CEREBRAL PALSY - CURRENT STEPS

Edited by **Mintaze Kerem Gunel**

Cerebral Palsy - Current Steps
http://dx.doi.org/10.5772/61951
Edited by Mintaze Kerem Gunel

Contributors

Emine Eda Kurt, Pedro Diz-Dios, Maite Abeleira Pazos, Mercedes Outumuro, Marcio Diniz-Freitas, Lucia García-Caballero, Jacobo Limeres, Ayşe Numanoğlu Akbaş, Deepak Sharan, Joshua Samuel Rajkumar, Rajarajeshwari Balakrishnan, Amruta Kulkarni, Alejandro Ramirez, Mauro José Conte, Cleiton Eduardo Saturno, Mísia Farhat, Elaine Carmelita Piucco, Fabiana De Melo Giacomini Garcez Garcez, Ana Carolina Savall, Nilay Çömük Balcı, Özge Çankaya, Kübra Seyhan, Cemil Ozal, Duygu Turker, Duygu Korkem

Published by InTech

Janeza Trdine 9, 51000 Rijeka, Croatia

Publishing Process Manager Andrea Koric

Technical Editor SPi Global

Cover InTech Design team

First published September, 2016

Printed in Croatia

Additional hard copies can be obtained from orders@intechopen.com

Cerebral Palsy - Current Steps, Edited by Mintaze Kerem Gunel

p. cm.

Print ISBN 978-953-51-2648-5
Online ISBN 978-953-51-2649-2

For EU product safety concerns:
IN TECH d.o.o., Prolaz Marije Krucifikse Kozulić 3, 51000 Rijeka, Croatia,
info@intechopen.com or visit our website at intechopen.com.

Meet the editor

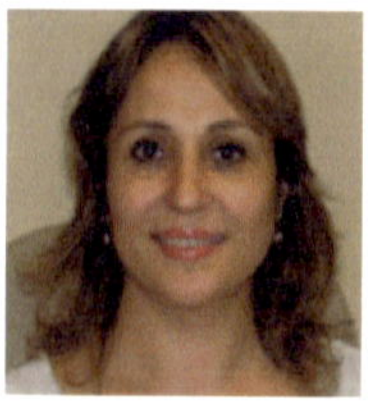

Professor Mintaze Kerem Günel, PT, PhD, graduated from Hacettepe University, School of Physical Therapy and Rehabilitation in 1989. In the same year, she began to work in Hacettepe University Hospital, Department of Physical Therapy and Rehabilitation, as a physiotherapist. She received her doctorate degree supported by Hacettepe University Research Bursary in 1998. Currently, she is teaching "Pediatric Rehabilitation" lessons for graduate students of physiotherapy. This lesson includes physiotherapy approaches and applications in children with risky babies, cerebral palsy, congenital torticollis, meningomyelocele, obstetric brachial plexus palsy, developmental disorders, and allied neurologic and developmental problems of children. Since 1993, she is a member of the European Academy of Childhood Disability (EACD) and the country representative of Turkey as well. She is an EBTA tutor in 2012 for Bobath training children and adults with cerebral palsy. She is a chairwoman of the Association of Child Physiotherapists and Neurodevelopmental Therapists. She is teaching pediatric rehabilitation for the students with graduate and postgraduate (doctorate and master's degree) level as a lecturer and as a professor.

Contents

Preface IX

Section 1 Definition, Epidemiology and Etiological Factors of Cerebral Palsy 1

Chapter 1 **Definition, Epidemiology, and Etiological Factors of Cerebral Palsy 3**
Emine Eda Kurt

Section 2 Evaluation 21

Chapter 2 **Assessments and Outcome Measures of Cerebral Palsy 23**
Ayşe Numanoğlu Akbaş

Section 3 Therapies 49

Chapter 3 **Current Rehabilitation Methods for Cerebral Palsy 51**
Nilay Çömük Balcı

Chapter 4 **ICF-CY-Based Physiotherapy Management in Children with Cerebral Palsy 79**
Özge Çankaya and Kübra Seyhan

Chapter 5 **Strength Training in People with Cerebral Palsy 103**
Cemil Özal, Duygu Türker and Duygu Korkem

Section 4 Interventions 127

Chapter 6 **Orthodontic Treatment in Children with Cerebral Palsy 129**
María Teresa Abeleira, Mercedes Outumuro, Marcio Diniz, Lucía García-Caballero, Pedro Diz and Jacobo Limeres

Chapter 7 **Neuromusculoskeletal Rehabilitation of Severe Cerebral Palsy 141**
Deepak Sharan, Joshua Samuel Rajkumar, Rajarajeshwari Balakrishnan and Amruta Kulkarni

Chapter 8 **Assistive and Adaptive Technology in Cerebral Palsy 173**
Alejandro Rafael Garcia Ramirez, Cleiton Eduardo Saturno, Mauro José Conte, Jéferson Fernandes da Silva, Mísia Farhat, Fabiana de Melo Giacomini Garcez Garcez, Ana Carolina Savall and Elaine Carmelita Piucco

Preface

Cerebral palsy (CP), the most common cause of physical disability in children, is a nonprogressive neurological impairment that is a result of an injury in the developing brain and it causes various neuromuscular and cognitive disabilities. CP is often accompanied by other disturbances of sensation, cognition, communication, perception, and behavior and seizure problems. It also leads to multiple problems that affect functionality and psychosocial health of children and adolescents, so they are unable to play important roles in their family, school, and other environments. Thus, rehabilitation aims to improve functional health status and increase independence in daily life, school, and social environment, which are very crucial for the CP treatment. Rehabilitation of the child with CP is difficult, often frustrating, and sometimes depressing. This is even more pronounced in countries with limited resources for the handicapped. An interdisciplinary management approach is the only means to integrate children with CP.

I would like to thank our book company InTech and all authors. I am indebted to Ms. Andrea Korić for helping us with text editing of this book.

I hope readers will benefit from our book and they will use this book in their treatment and clinical decision.

Mintaze Kerem Gunel, PT, PhD, Prof.
Hacettepe University, Faculty of Health Sciences,
Department of Physiotherapy and Rehabilitation,
Cerebral Palsy and pediatric Physiotherapy Unit,
Ankara, Turkey

Section 1

Definition, Epidemiology and Etiological Factors of Cerebral Palsy

Chapter 1

Definition, Epidemiology, and Etiological Factors of Cerebral Palsy

Emine Eda Kurt

Additional information is available at the end of the chapter

http://dx.doi.org/10.5772/64768

Abstract

CP is not a diagnosis but an "umbrella term for many clinical descriptions. It refers to a group of permanent disorders of the development of movement and posture, causing activity limitation, that are attributed to nonprogressive disturbances that occurred in the developing fetal or infant brain. The motor disorerders of cerebral palsy are often accompanied by disturbances of sensation, perception, cognition. First description was made in 19th century by William Little. CP prevalence is generally reported around 2-3 per 1000 live births in both developed and developing countries (even if for very different reasons). Additionally for term children CP prevalence is 1 per 1000 live births. This rates are 6-10 times higher in preterm birth. The etiology of CP has been reported very diverse and multifactorial as prenatal, perinatal and postnatal. The causes and risk factors are congenital, genetic, inflammatory, infectious, anoxic, traumatic and metabolic. Knowledge of the epidemiology and etiology of cerebral palsy is important. Thus, at least in some cases, early diagnosis and prevention can be achieved.

Keywords: Cerebral Palsy, Definition, Epidemiology, Etiology, Risk factors

1. Definition

Cerebral palsy (CP) is a well-recognized neurodevelopmental condition beginning in early childhood and persisting throughout the lifetime. It was first reported by William little, who was an orthopedic surgeon, in 1843 as cerebral paresis [1, 2]. Little focused on joint contractures and deformities resulting from long-standing spasticity and paralysis. Additionally, he indicated that the cause of the spasticity and paralysis was often due to damage to the brain during infancy and, specifically, preterm birth and perinatal asphyxia [3].

The most comprehensive study until then was published in 1862 by William Little. The association between a large number of patients' clinical presentation and their birth history as recalled by the family was described in this study. Little differentiated between the congenital deformities observed at the time of birth, such as talipes equinovarus, and the limb deformities that developed subsequently to preterm, difficult, or traumatic births, which he termed as spastic rigidity. It was described as a disorder that appeared to strike children in the first year of life, affected developmental skill progression, and did not improve over time [4].

Then, Sarah McNutt described that it continued to raise the profile of the risks of long-term disability arising from birth trauma [5]. At the end of the nineteenth century, Sigmund Freud suggested that CP might be rooted in the brain's development in the womb and related aberrant development to factors influencing the developing fetus [2, 6, 7]. In addition, in the early 1920s, some 30 years after Freud's comments, an American orthopedic surgeon made the next major contribution for understanding of CP [8].

In the twentieth century, newer documented concepts of cerebral palsy have been defined. Mac Keith and Polani [1, 8] described CP as "a persisting but not unchanging disorder of movement and posture, occurring in the early years of life due to a nonprogressive disorder of the brain, the result of interference during its development." In 1964, Bax [9] reported a description of CP suggested by an international working group that has become a classic and is still used. It was expressed that CP is a disorder of movement and posture due to a defect or lesion of the immature brain. Although this definition is usually all that is cited by authors, some additional comments were added by Bax: "For practical purposes it is usual to exclude from cerebral palsy those disorders of posture and movement which are of short duration, due to progressive disease or due solely to mental deficiency." Bax and his group felt that this simple sentence can be readily translated into other languages and hoped that it may be used universally. At that time, it was felt wiser not to define completely what they meant by immature brain, as any such description may be restricted services to those in need. Like its predecessors, this formulation of the CP concept placed an exclusive focus on motor aspects and also stressed the specific consequences of early as opposed to late-acquired brain damage. It was not formally included in the concept that cognitive, sensory, behavioral, and other associated impairments were very prevalent in people with disordered movement and posture due to a defect or lesion of the immature brain, a frequent significant disability. This definition continued to emphasize the motor impairment and acknowledged its variability, previously underscored in the MacKeith and Polani definition; it also excluded progressive disease, a point introduced in Bax's annotation [8]. The heterogeneity of disorders covered by the term of CP, as well as advances in understanding of development in infants with early brain damage, led Mutch et al. [10] to modify the definition of CP in 1992 as follows: an umbrella term covering a group of nonprogressive, but often changing, motor impairment syndromes secondary to lesions or anomalies of the brain arising in the early stages of development.

To underline the idea that a comprehensive approach to CP needs to be multidimensional and that management of patients with CP almost always requires a multidisciplinary setting, classes of disorders commonly accompanying CP have been identified and included in the revised definition [1]. And last definition of CP, which is comprised to prior assessments and

http://dx.doi.org/10.5772/64768

identifications, was made in April 2006. CP describes a group of persistent disorders of the development of movement and posture causing activity limitations that are attributed to nonprogressive disturbances that occurred in the developing fetal or infant brain. The motor disorders of cerebral palsy are often accompanied by disturbances of sensation, perception, cognition, communication, and behavior by epilepsy and secondary musculoskeletal problems. This description was authored by the members of the executive committee functioning in panels enriched with expertise from consultants and by comments and suggestions from many reviewers responding to drafts provided to the international community. It is offered for international consensus and adoption, with the intent of providing a broad spectrum of audiences with a common conceptualization about cerebral palsy [1]. CP is defined as a group of nonprogressive, but often changing, motor impairment syndromes secondary to lesions or abnormalities of the brain and emerging in the early stages of development [10]. CP is a symptom complex rather than a disease. It is a concept derived from an insult to a growing, developing brain and therefore it is a dynamic changing clinical picture emanating from static pathology [11]. CP may be diagnosed during the first two years of life, especially when functional impairment is mild [12, 13].

This specification contains the concept that CP is a group of neurodevelopmental disorders that involve numerous developing functions. As in other neurodevelopmental disorders, various manifestations of the disordered brain may appear more significantly in different persons or at different life periods, e.g., some aspects of the motor impairment, sensory loss, attentional difficulty, epilepsy, musculoskeletal dysfunction, intellectual disability, and many others maybe more prominent or more problematic at different periods of the life of a person with CP [1].

In 2010, Blair again emphasized that CP is not a diagnosis but an “umbrella term for many clinical descriptions.” It has covered a wide variety of clinical conditions that meet the following four criteria:

- The presence of a disorder of movement or posture.

- Secondary to a cerebral abnormality.

- Arising early in development.

- By the time movement impairment exists, the cerebral abnormality is static.

There is no test, genetic, metabolic, immunologic, or otherwise, that demonstrates the existence or absence of CP because there is no specified cause, cerebral pathology, or even type of motor impairment resulting from nonprogressive cerebral pathology acquired early in life. Even as a clinical description, these criteria fail in several aspects to achieve the precision required of a definition [14, 15]. For example, specifying the age at which development is no longer considered “early.” There is no agreement on this age [16].

Because it is difficult to definitively differentiate between pre- and neonatally acquired brain damage, all those not postneonatally acquired are usually considered together. The four criteria cannot be addressed until (a) motor development can be clearly recognized as being normal or disordered and (b) the possibility of progressive cerebral disease can be excluded.

Signs suggesting disordered motor control may be recognized very early in life, but accurate prediction has only been confirmed by trained observers in the small proportion of persons with CP born very preterm [17]. Acquisition of the cerebral abnormality may precede recognition of the motor disorder by many months or even years. However, brain-impaired infants, particularly the most severely impaired, are at increased risk of dying before reaching an age at which the criteria for CP can be confirmed. Early death is a competing outcome. On the other hand, it is difficult to definitively exclude the possibility of progression or resolution at any age. Even if cerebral pathology is static, motor abilities change in all children over time, even if that development is grossly abnormal, making functional change an unreliable marker for progressive cerebral pathology. Conversely, a proportion of children described as CP at an early age catch up with their normally developing peers at a later age [18]. Therefore, the choice of an age that must be attained before being counted as CP, as well as the age beyond which development is no longer early, is arbitrary and depends on the interest in using the CP label. Treating clinicians are more flexible in applying the CP label because their primary concern is to balance the psychological effects of labeling a child having CP with the therapeutic opportunities that the label can afford. This balance can change with time. Registers with a long lifespan require primarily a constant definition over time, and this was the guiding principle of the recommendation by Badawi et al. [19] that conditions historically excluded from CP (not "diagnosed" as CP on account of having another diagnosis) continue to be excluded, even if meeting the criteria for CP. By contrast, reliability between current observers is the guiding principle of the more recent multicenter surveillance system in Europe, which adopted a flowchart to decision inclusion or exclusion of cases of cerebral palsy on registration [20]. However, the reality of barriers to achieving interobserver agreement of classification is demonstrated by the relatively poor agreement achieved with this flowchart [21]. Diagnosis of CP is not easy. It needs time to be confirmed. Premature diagnosis leading to over-ascertainment (because of transient anomalies in preterm babies) or under-ascertainment, as stated above, is not an unchanging condition with the clinical aspect in some cases altering as a child develops. There is consensus that 5 years of age was the optimal age for confirmation of diagnosis [22].

2. Epidemiology

CP prevalence is usually reported around 2–3 per 1000 live births in both developed and developing countries for very different reasons [23, 24]. For term children, CP prevalence is 1 per 1000 live births. Additionally, for moderately preterm children (32–36 weeks' gestation), forecasts are 6–10 times higher and for very preterm children (less than 32 weeks' gestation), prevalence is 10 times higher than the moderately preterm children. CP rates for live births show a lower prevalence for babies of birthweight less than 1000 g than for those with a birthweight of 1000–1499 g. This paradoxical effect is caused from the high number of babies who do not live long enough to develop CP and it disappears when forecasting prevalence for neonatal survivors. Changes in perinatal and neonatal mortality accelerated in most countries from the 1960s, with a huge decrease up until the late 1980s, when there was an increase in the absolute number of children with CP. From 1990s, there has been a plateauing of mortality rates but a downward trend in CP rates, mainly in moderate and very low birthweight (VLBW) children. In most studies, the CP rates in children born at term or with normal birthweight seem rather stable over time. This finding is especially relevant since normal birthweight and term children represent at least one-half of children with CP and, thus, it may be connected to the persisting stagnation of CP prevalence, despite continuous improvement in perinatal care and in mortality rates [25–27].

There were different rates of CP reported in recent five decades from different population. Published rates from geographically defined populations show significant differences, primarily due to variations in methods (**Table 1**). Variations within a reporting system over time tend to be smaller [28].

The proportion of children described as CP increases with decreasing gestational age at birth. The advent of mechanical ventilation to neonatal intensive care has allowed survival of increasingly preterm births, creating a new source of high-risk neonates and perhaps a new cause of brain damage [27].

Area	Year range	Number of cases	Rate of per 1000
Turkey [29–31]	1990–2006	186	4.4
	1988–2003	102	1.1
	1990–1995		5.5
Sweden [32]	1995–1998	170	1.9
Canada [33]	1991–1995		2.7
U.S.A. [34]	2002	416	3.6
Australia [35]	1970–1998	2950	1.61
	1970–1972		1.4
	1996–1998		1.4
United Kingdom [36]	1984–2002	1301	2.0
	1984–1988		2.5
	1999–2001		1.2
Norway [37]	1996–1998	374	2.1
Danimark [38]	1971–1974		1.7
	1975–1978		1.6
	1979–1982		2.6
	1983–1986		3.0
	1987–1990		2.4
France [39]	1980–1989	261	1.78

Table 1. Published rates of CP from population-based samples.

3. Etiological factors

The etiology of CP is very diverse and multifactorial. The causes are congenital, genetic, inflammatory, infectious, anoxic, traumatic, and metabolic. The injury to the developing brain may be prenatal, natal, or postnatal [40]. Due to the lack of a definitive test for CP, multiple and different possible causes also constitute a challenge in this context. For more than 30% of children, there are no risk factors or known etiology [41, 42] but some risk factors have repeatedly been observed to be related to CP [43]. CP may result from one or more etiologies and can occur at any stage from before conception to infancy, with the actual cause difficult to determine in all cases [41, 42, 44]. Known causes according to the timing of the brain insult can be classified, respectively, as prenatal, perinatal, and postnatal.

3.1. Prenatal causes of cerebral palsy

Among the important known causes of cerebral palsy are congenital brain malformations including malformations of cortical development. Modern imaging techniques enable more children with these conditions to be identified [45, 46]. Currently, problems occurring during intrauterine development, congenital disorders, asphyxia occurring in any gestational age, and preterm birth are thought to account for the majority of cases [47]. Neuroimaging studies support the current thought that prenatal causes of CP, such as brain malformations, intrauterine vascular malformations, and infection, are more common than birth asphyxia [48]. Although intrapartum asphyxia was originally thought to be a major reason for CP, it accounts for only 10–20% of cases. The most frequent perinatal or neonatal etiologies in low birthweight infants are periventricular leukomalacia (PVL), periventricular hemorrhage, and cerebral infarction, but in infants of normal birthweight, the most common reason is hypoxicischemic encephalopathy. Knowledge about the cortical dysplasias, of which some have a genetic basis, is increasing rapidly [49]. Periventricular leukomalacia is a risk factor with 60–100% of patients with PVL developing CP. In general, congenital malformations are strongly associated with cerebral palsy [50–54]. Other known antenatal causes of cerebral palsy are vascular events demonstrated by brain imaging (for example, middle cerebral artery occlusion), and maternal TORCH (toxoplasmosis, rubella, cytomegalovirus, and herpes simplex) infections during the first and second trimesters of pregnancy are the known causes of long-term neurodevelopmental disabilities. In industrialized countries, the proportion of CP attributable to TORCH infections is estimated to be almost 5% [13]. The less common causes of cerebral palsy include metabolic disorders, maternal ingestion of toxins, and rare genetic syndromes [55].

3.2. Perinatal causes

Antepartum hemorrhage, obstructed labor, or cord prolapse can jeopardize the fetus causing hypoxia, but essential criteria must be fulfilled before cerebral palsy can be attributed to the acute intrapartum period [56, 57]. These criteria are metabolic acidosis in umbilical arterial cord, fetal scalp or very early neonatal blood samples, and early onset of severe or moderate neonatal encephalopathy in infants of >34 weeks gestation [57].

Children with cerebral palsy, who have a history of neonatal encephalopathy, are more likely to have had signs of intrapartum hypoxia such as meconium staining of the amniotic fluid [58]. However, there may be no evidence of perinatal asphyxia in a significant percentage of children with neonatal encephalopathy [19]. In a systematic study, cerebral palsy was more strongly associated with encephalopathy [59]. Severe hypoglycaemia, untreated jaundice, and severe neonatal infection in neonatal period may be responsible for cerebral palsy [55].

3.3. Postnatal causes

Infection and injuries are responsible for most cases of postneonatally acquired cerebral palsy in developed countries. Thanks to introduction of new vaccines, meningitis and subsequent neurological sequelae were decreased in a large number of children. Accidental (motor vehicle accidents and near-drowning episodes) and nonaccidental injuries may responsible for cerebral palsy. Other reasons of postneonatally acquired cerebral palsy contain apparent life-threatening events, cerebrovascular accidents, and following surgery for congenital malformations. Meningitis, septicemia, malaria, and other conditions are the important causes of cerebral palsy in developing countries [55].

The risk factors associated with CP may also be presented as maternal, paternal and sibling factors, prenatal factors, perinatal factors, and postnatal factors.

3.4. Maternal, paternal, and sibling factors

Maternal medical conditions are associated with cerebral palsy. These include intellectual disability, seizures [60], maternal thrombophilia [33], and thyroid disease [50, 60]; prior reproductive loss [61] and CP in a sibling have been reported as an association with CP in the Collaborative Perinatal Project of the National Institute of Neurological and Communicative Disorders and Stroke [60]. Adolescent pregnants are likely to have low gestational weeks, low birthweight, and birth traumas. Maternal age > 35 years was reported among risk factors of CP [13]. Öztürk et al. [30] also reported that mothers of children with CP were significantly younger, with an increase in adolescent pregnancies. Mothers of children with CP had low gestational weeks, low birthweight, and prolonged labor.

Parental consanguinity [62, 63] and low economic status were found related to CP in two studies [64, 65].

3.5. Prenatal risk factors

Preeclampsia is associated with an increased risk of cerebral palsy in term infants [66] but this association does not seem to exist in preterm infants [67, 68]. It has been suggested that preeclampsia may lead to a release of catecholamines in preterm infants, which accelerates fetal maturation [69], but care is needed in comparing rates in infants of the same gestation, given that preeclampsia itself can be directly responsible for preterm births. Alternatively, the presence of preeclampsia may result in elective preterm delivery, avoiding the inflammatory responses of spontaneous preterm labors with all their associated problems.

Chorioamnionitis and intrauterine infection and/or inflammation are well-known risk factors for CP. Prenatal maternal chorioamnionitis is accounting for as much as 12% of cerebral palsy in term infants and 28% in premature infants [13, 70, 71]. According to the inflammatory hypothesis, maternal infection can lead to elevated fetal blood and brain cytokine levels, which might result in central nervous damage and subsequent CP [13]. Nelson et al. reported that blood inflammatory cytokine levels in term infants that developed CP were significantly higher than control groups [72]. A number of studies have shown that even fever itself might be harmful. There may be toxic products of the infecting organisms or toxic effects of inflammatory mediators produced by the mother, infant, or placenta. It is tempting to consider that cytokines or other inflammatory mediators induced brain damage directly or indirectly [73, 74]. Gilles et al. [75] demonstrated that maternal trauma in pregnancy may be implicated as a possible cause of cerebral palsy. Antepartum hemorrhage is also associated with mortality, CP, and white matter damage in preterm infants [76].

Multiple pregnancies, also reported as a risk factor of CP, increase fourfold in twins and 18-fold in triplets [77]. These are associated with preterm delivery, poor intrauterine growth, birth defects, and intrapartum complications [78, 79].

Intrauterine growth restriction (IUGR) can be responsible to increase risk of neonatal morbidity and mortality, and also seems to affect brain development [80]. In some specific variance in the brain of IUGR infants, as restriction of the volume of gray matter, a reduced amount of the total DNA in glia cells and neurons, and changes in cerebral hemodynamic have been reported. This hypothesis supported by animal studies showed reduced oxygen delivery to the brain and retarded growth of the forebrain and cerebellum [81, 82]. Several mechanisms have been suggested for the relation between IUGR in term babies and CP. The abnormal growth may play a direct role in causing CP or utero brain injury. Alternatively, a separate process, such as placental insufficiency, could cause both the growth retardation and brain injury [83, 84].

Two mutations have been detected, which predispose heterozygous carriers to venous thrombosis. One is a mutation localized to the factor V gene (factor V Leiden mutation, VL) and second is the gene for prothrombin [85, 86]. Nelson et al. reported that placental thrombosis, or neonatal stroke, may have occurred and resulted in CP [72].

Males are at higher risk of CP, perhaps because of the recently identified gender-specific neuronal vulnerabilities [15, 87]. In the fetus, CP has been associated with intrauterine growth restriction [88, 89] maternal factors [90, 91], other risk factors [92], and congenital anomalies not only of the brain, head, eyes, and face, but also with noncerebral anomalies (in the apparent absence of cerebral anomalies), particularly of the heart, limbs, and skeleton [93, 94]. The risk of CP also increases with the number of suboptimal factors affecting a pregnancy [50, 95].

3.6. Perinatal risk factors

According to the results of World Health Report, perinatal asphyxia and high-risk pregnancy were independent factors that correlated with CP in term and near-term newborns. In developing countries, 4–9 million infants experience birth asphyxia annually [96]. Major events likely to cause perinatal asphyxia include prolonged delivery, breech delivery, and emergency cesarean births [54, 97]. Though intrapartum factors producing asphyxia were traditionally accepted to be the principal cause of CP, this assumption was reconsidered during the 1980s and 1990s, and today it is suggested that 70–80% of cases of CP are due to prenatal factors and that birth asphyxia plays a relatively minor role. Although intrapartum asphyxia is believed to account for around 10% of CP in term and near-term infants, Swedish population-based CP report by the Hagberg group detected birth asphyxia to be the likely cause of CP in 28% of term children with CP [98]. However, "birth asphyxia" is a poorly defined term related to a sequence initiated by hypoxia and its clinical signs are nonspecific [43]. Using indirect signs of birth asphyxia, recent studies suggest that birth asphyxia might not be such an important cause of CP as was previously assumed, but that it might sometimes constitute one element of a multifactorial cause; neonatal signs associated with birth asphyxia might be early manifestations of CP from a variety of causes, of which birth asphyxia is only one; and the majority of pathways to CP commence antenatally [13, 43, 99]. Any factor causing a very preterm birth that lies on a potential causal path to CP must be remembered. Many etiologic studies control or stratify the risk of CP that also increases with the number of suboptimal factors affecting a pregnancy [100].

The lower birthweights and shorter gestations associated with multiple birth contribute significantly to their higher risk of CP, but cannot be the only relevant factors because gestation-specific rates are higher for multiples than for singletons born at term or extremely preterm [101, 102]. The most important risk factor seems to be prematurity, and low birthweight with risk of CP increasing with decreasing gestational age and birthweight. About 28% of CP cases are born very preterm, compared to 1% of all births. As an effect of the success of neonatal intensive care during the last three decades, ensuring an increasing survival of children born extremely preterm, the prevalence of CP among preterm children has risen [103]. These groups of children may contribute significantly to the overall number of children with CP since they are at greater risk of developing CP. Although it can be expected that where mortality rates are high and CP rates are low, It may be that thanks to good clinical practice and developing technology mortality and CP prevalence rate will be reduced. Neonatal intensive care practices, including withdrawal of life support, may have an impact on local CP rates over time; this influence is difficult to assess [13, 104].

Abruptio placentae have also been suggested to be associated with a higher risk of CP, especially moderately preterm (32–36 weeks) groups [105]. Perinatal infections (bacterial, viral, and protozoal) may also cause the development of CP [106].

Other relations with cerebral palsy include prolonged rupture of the membranes in infants of all gestations [52] and in preterm babies [67]; the presence of meconium-stained fluid [107] and tight nuchal cord was also reported as associated with CP [108].

3.7. Postnatal risk factors of CP

Postneonatally acquired CP is said to result from a recognized brain damaging event that is unrelated to factors in the antenatal or perinatal period, but there is a growing realization that the pathway to postneonatally acquired CP often begins before the postneonatal period [19]. The inclusion criteria for a postneonatal time range of the insult vary between reports. Some researchers have included cases acquired from neonatal causes that might have had their origin during pregnancy, labor, or delivery [109]. Although a strict definition of beyond 28 days is used by others [16], the upper age limit also varied from 2 to 10 years between researchers [110]. Population-based estimates of the frequency of postneonatally acquired CP, as a proportion of all CP, are reported in the literature to change between 1.4 and 24%, with higher rates in undeveloped and developing countries, and lower socio-economic groups [16]. The Surveillance of Cerebral Palsy in Europe, in a cohort of children from eight countries born between 1976 and 1990, reported that the rate of children whose CP was of postneonatal origin was 7.8% [39]. Pharoah et al. suggested that postnatal causes are generally resulted in spastic CP [111]. Most surveillance systems distinguish cases in which motor impairment is obviously acquired postneonatally, usually following cerebral infection or head trauma [16]. Other infection complications, cerebrovascular accidents, trauma, hypoxia, gastroenteritis, and other causes of acute encephalopathy, neoplasmas, and exposure toxins were other reasons that are reported [112]. Infection, however, remains an important cause of acquired CP despite a fall in the overall numbers more than 30 years of the study. With the introduction of new vaccines, the proportion of cases due to infection will be further decrease, providing there is adequate education and regular control [16].

CP is a nonprogressive but permanent disorder. The disease has been better understood by the researchers in due course of time, and then described as "CP is not a diagnosis but an umbrella term." Though there are different rates according to the region, percentage of CP is not low in especially developing and undeveloped countries. Etiological factors of CP are very diverse and may be classified according to time period (prenatal, perinatal, postneonatal) and parenteral factors. It may be that, thanks to good clinical practice and developing technology, the prevalence of CP rate will be reduced and additionally most known risk factors will be avoided.

Author details

Emine Eda Kurt

Address all correspondence to: eedakurt@gmail.com

Ahi Evran University, Medical Faculty, Department of Physical Medicine and Rehabilitation, Kırşehir, Turkey

References

[1] Rosenbaum P, Paneth N, Leviton A, Goldstein M, Bax M, et al. A report: the definition and classification of cerebral palsy April 2006. Dev Med Child Neurol Suppl 2007;109:8–14.

[2] Morris C. Definition and classification of cerebral palsy: a historical perspective. Dev Med Child Neurol 2007;49(109):3–7.

[3] Little WJ. Lectures on the deformity of the human frame. Lancet 1843;1:318–320.

[4] Little WJ. On the incidence of abnormal parturition, difficult labour, premature birth and asphyxia neonatorurn on the mental and physical condition of the child, especially in relation to deformities. Trans Obstetr Soc London 1862;3:293–344.

[5] McNutt SJ. Apoplexia neonatorum. Am J Obstetr 1885;1:73.

[6] Freud S. Les diplegies cerebrales infantiles. Rev Neurol 1893;1:177–183.

[7] Accardo PJ. Freud on diplegia: commentary and translation. Am J Dis Child 1982;136:452–456.

[8] Mac Keith RC, Polani PE. The little club: memorandum on terminology and classification of cerebral palsy. Cerebral Palsy Bull 1959;5:27–35.

[9] Bax MCO. Terminology and classification of cerebral palsy. Dev Med Child Neurol 1964;l6:295–307.

[10] Mutch LW, Alberman E, Hagberg B, Kodama K, Velickovic MV. Cerebral palsy epidemiology: where are we now and where are we going? Dev Med Child Neurol 1992;34:547–555.

[11] Brown K. Cerebral palsy: can we prevent it? Dev Med Child Neurol Suppl 2003;95:30.

[12] Ford GW, Kitchen WH, Doyle LW, et al. Changing diagnosis of cerebral palsy in very low birthweight children. Am J Perinatol 1990;7(2):178–181.

[13] Jacobsson B, Hagberg G. Antenatal risk factors for cerebral palsy. Best Pract Res Clin Obstet Gynaecol 2004;18(3):425–436.

[14] Blair E, Love S. Commentary on the definition and classification of cerebral palsy. Dev Med Child Neurol 2005;47:510.

[15] Stanley F, Blair E, Alberman E. 'What are the cerebral palsies?' Cerebral Palsies: Epidemiology and Causal Pathways. London: MacKeith Press; 2000;pp. 8–13, Chapter 2.

[16] Reid S, Lanigan A, Reddihough D. Post-neonatally acquired cerebral palsy in Victoria, Australia, 1970–1999. J Paediatr Child Health 2006;42(10):606–611.

[17] Constantinou J, Adamson-Macedo E, Mirmiran M, et al. Movement, imaging and neurobehavioural assessment as predictors of cerebral palsy in preterm infants. J Perinatol 2007;27(4):225–229.

[18] Nelson KB, Ellenberg JH. Children who 'outgrew' cerebral palsy. Pediatrics 1982;69(5): 529–536.

[19] Badawi N, Watson L, Petterson B, et al. What constitutes cerebral palsy? Dev Med Child Neurol 1998;40:520–527.

[20] Surveillance of Cerebral Palsy in Europe (SCPE) Surveillance of cerebral palsy in Europe: a collaboration of cerebral palsy surveys and registers. Dev Med Child Neurol. 2000;42(12):816–824.

[21] Gainsborough M, Surman G, Maestri G, Colver A, Cans C. Validity and reliability of the guidelines of the surveillance of cerebral palsy in Europe for the classification of cerebral palsy. Dev Med Child Neurol 2008;50(11):828–831.

[22] Cans C, Dolk H, Platt MJ, et al. Recommendations from the SCPE collaborative group for defining and classifying cerebral palsy. Dev Med Child Neurol 2007;49(109):35–38.

[23] Nelson KB. Can we prevent cerebral palsy? N Engl J Med 2003;349:1765–1769.

[24] Kadhim H, Sébire G, Kahn A, Evrard P, Dan B. Causal mechanisms underlying periventricular leukomalacia and cerebral palsy. Curr Pediatr Rev 2005;1:1–6.

[25] Tu J, Willison D, Silver F, et al. Impracticality of informed consent in the registry of the Canadian Stroke Network. N Engl J Med 2004;350:1414–1421.

[26] Ingelfinger J, Drazen J. Registry research and medical privacy. N Engl J Med 2004;350(14):1452.

[27] Aly H. Mechanical ventilation and cerebral palsy. Pediatrics 2005;115(6):1765–1766.

[28] Blair E. Epidemiology of the cerebral palsies. Orthopedic Clinics of North America 2010;41(4):441-455.

[29] Serdaroglu A, Cansu A, Özkan S, Tezcan S. Prevalence of cerebral palsy in Turkish children between the ages of 2 and 16 years. Dev Med Child Neurol 2006;48(6):413–416.

[30] Öztürk A, Demirci F, Yavuz T, et al. Antenatal and delivery risk factors and prevalence of cerebral palsy in Duzce (Turkey). Brain Dev 2007;29(1):39–42.

[31] Okan N, Okan M, Eralp O, Aytekin AH. The prevalence of neurological disorders among children in Gemlik (Turkey). Dev Med Child Neurol 1995;37(7):597–603.

[32] Himmelmann K, Hagberg G, Beckung E, et al. The changing panorama of cerebral palsy in Sweden. IX. Prevalence and origin in the birth-year period 1995–1998. Acta Paediatr 2005;94:287–294.

[33] Smith L, Kelly K, Prkachin G, et al. The prevalence of cerebral palsy in British Columbia, 1991–1995. Can J Neurol Sci 2008;35(3):342–347.

[34] Yeargin-Allsopp M, Van Naarden Braun K, Doernberg N, et al. Prevalence of cerebral palsy in 8-year-old children in three areas of the United States in 2002: a multisite collaboration. Pediatrics 2008;121(3):547–554.

[35] Reid SM, Lanigan A, Walstab JE, et al. The Victorian Cerebral Palsy Register. Melbourne, Australia: Murdoch Childrens' Research Institute; 2005.

[36] Surman G, Newdick H, King A, Gallagher M, Kurinczuk JJ. Child: four counties database of cerebral palsy, vision loss, and hearing loss in children. Annual report 2008: including data for births 1984 to 2002. Oxford, UK: National Perinatal Epidemiology Unit; 2008.

[37] Andersen G, Irgens L, Haagaas I, et al. Cerebral palsy in Norway: prevalence, subtypes and severity. Eur J Paediatr Neurol 2008;12(1):4–13.

[38] Uldall P, Michelsen SI, Topp M, Madsen M. The Danish cerebral palsy registry. Dan Med Bull 2001;48: 161–163.

[39] Surveillance of cerebral palsy in Europe (SCPE). Prevalence and characteristics of children with cerebral palsy in Europe. Dev Med Child Neurol 2002;44(9):633–640.

[40] Sankar C, Mundkur N. Cerebral palsy—definition, classification, etiology and early diagnosis. Indian J Pediatr 2005;72(10):865–868.

[41] Taft LT. Accentuating the positive for children with cerebral palsy. Except Parent 1999;29:64–66.

[42] Rosembaum P. Cerebral palsy: what parents and doctors want to know. Brit Med J 2003;326:970–974.

[43] Blair E, Stanley F. Issues in the classification and epidemiology of cerebral palsy. Mental Retard Dev Disabil Res Rev 2002;3:184–193.

[44] Jones MW, Morgan E, Shelton CE, Thorogood C. Cerebral palsy: introduction and diagnosis (Part I). J Pediatr Health Care 2007;21:146–152.

[45] Krageloh-Mann I, Petersen D, Hagberg G, Vollmer B, Hagberg B, Michaelis R. Bilateral spastic cerebral palsy—MRI pathology and origin: analysis from a representative series of 56 cases. Dev Med Child Neurol 1995;37:379–397.

[46] Steinlin M, Good M, Martin E, Banziger O, Largo RH, Boltshauser E. Congenital hemiplegia: morphology of cerebral lesions and pathogenetic aspects from MRI. Neuropediatrics 1993;24:224–229.

[47] Moster D, Lie R, Irgens L, Bjerkedal T, Markestad T. The association of Apgar score with subsequent death and cerebral palsy: a population-based study in term infants. J Pediatr 2001;138:798–803.

[48] Truwit CL, Barkovich AJ, Koch TK, Ferriero DM. Cerebral palsy: MR findings in 40 patients. Am J Neuroradiol 1992;13:67–78.

[49] Dobyns WB, Truwit CL. Lissencephaly and other malformations of cortical development: 1995 update. Neuropediatrics 1995;26:132–147.

[50] Blair E, Stanley F. Etiological pathways to spastic cerebral palsy. Paediatr Perinatal Epidemiol 1993;7:302–317.

[51] Croen L, Grether J, Curry C, Nelson K. Congenital abnormalities among children with cerebral palsy: more evidence for prenatal antecedents. J Pediatr 2001;138:804–812.

[52] Nelson KB, Ellenberg JH. Predictors of low and very low birth-weight and the relation of these to cerebral palsy. JAMA 1985;254:1473–1479.

[53] Palmer L, Blair E, Petterson B, Burton P. Antenatal antecedents of moderate and severe cerebral palsy. Paediatr Perinatal Epidemiol 1995;9:171–184.

[54] Torfs CP, van den Berg BJ, Oechsil FW, Cummins S. Prenatal and perinatal factors in the etiology of cerebral palsy. J Pediatr 1990;116:615–619.

[55] Reddihough DS, Collins KJ. The epidemiology and causes of cerebral palsy. Aust J Physiother 2003;49(1):7–12.

[56] Muraskas J, Ellsworth L, Culp E, Garbe G, Morrison J. Risk management in obstetrics and neonatal-perinatal medicine. In: Özdemir Ö (Ed). Complementary Pediatrics 2012, pp. 269–286. InTech, Available from: http://www.intechopen.com/books/complementary pediatrics/common allegations-of-professional-liability-against-practitioners-of-neonatal-perinatal-medicine; DOI: 10.5772/32846

[57] MacLennan A. For the international cerebral palsy task force: a template for defining a causal relation between acute intrapartum events and cerebral palsy: international consensus statement. BMJ 1999;319:1054–1059.

[58] Gaffney G, Flavell V, Johnston A, Squier M, Sellars S. Cerebral palsy and neonatal encephalopathy. Arch Dis Child 1994;70:195–200.

[59] Van de Riet JE, Vandenbussche FP, Le Cessie S, Keirse MJ. Newborn assessment and long-term adverse outcome: a systematic review. Am J Obstetr Gynaecol 1999;180:1024–1029.

[60] Nelson KB, Ellenberg JH. Antecedents of cerebral palsy. Multivariate analysis of risk factors. New Engl J Med 1986:315:81–86.

[61] Blair E, Stanley FJ. When can cerebral palsy be prevented? The generation of causal hypotheses by multivariate analysis of a case-control study. Paediatr Perinat Epidemiol 1993;7:272–301.

[62] Sinha G, Corry P, Subesinghe D, et al. Prevalence and type of cerebral palsy in a British ethnic community: the role of consanguinity. Dev Med Child Neurol 1997;39(4):259–262.

[63] Erkin G, Delialioglu S, Ozel S, et al. Risk factors and clinical profiles in Turkish children with cerebral palsy: analysis of 625 cases. Int J Rehabil Res 2008;31(1):89–91.

[64] Dowding VM, Barry C. Cerebral palsy: social class differences in prevalence in relation to birthweight and severity of disability. J Epidemiol Community Health 1990;44:191–195.

[65] Kramer MS, Goulet L, Lydon J, et al. Socio-economic disparities in preterm birth: causal pathways and mechanisms. Pediatr Perinatal Epidemiol 2001;15:104–123.

[66] Collins M, Paneth N. Pre-eclampsia and cerebral palsy: are they related? Dev Med Child Neurol 1988;40:207–211.

[67] Murphy DJ, Sellars S, MacKenzie IZ, Yudkin P, Johnson A. Case-control study of antenatal and intrapartum risk factors for cerebral palsy in very preterm singleton babies. Lancet 1995;346:1449–1454.

[68] Spinillo A, Capuzzo E, Cavallini A, Stronati M, De Santolo A, Fazzi E. Preeclampsia, preterm delivery and infant cerebral palsy. Eur J Obstetr Gynecol Reprod Biol 1998;7:151–155.

[69] Amiel-Tison C, Pettigrew C. Adaptive changes in the developing brain during intrauterine stress. Brain Dev 1991;13:67–76.

[70] Grether JK, Nelson KB, Walsh E, et al. Intrauterine exposure to infection and risk of cerebral palsy in very preterm infants. Arch Pediatr Adolescent Med 2003;157(1):26–32.

[71] Iliodromiti Z, Zygouris D, Karagianni P, et al. Brain injury in preterm infants. In: Raines D (Ed.). Neonatal Care 2012, pp. 73–86. Rijeka: InTech, Available from http://www.intechopen.com/books/neonatal-care/brain_injury_in_preterm_infants; DOI: 10.5772/52078

[72] Nelson KB, Dambrosia JM, Grether JK, Phillips TM. Neonatal cytokines and coagulation factors in children with cerebral palsy. Ann Neurol 1998;44(4):665–675.

[73] Nelson KB, Willoughby RE. Infection, inflammation and the risk of cerebral palsy. Curr Opin Neurol 2000;13(2):133–139.

[74] Nelson KB, Grether JK, Dambrosia JM, Dickens B, Phillips TM. Cytokine concentrations in neonatal blood of preterm children with cerebral palsy. Am J Obstet Gynecol 2000;182:47.

[75] Gilles MT, Blair E, Watson L, et al. Trauma in pregnancy and cerebral palsy: is there a link? MJA 1996;164:500–501.

[76] Stanley FJ, Blair E, Alberman E. Cerebral palsies: epidemiology and causal pathways. Clinics in Developmental Medicine. London: MacKeith Press; 2000. p. 151.

[77] Stanley F, Blair E, Alberman E. 'The special case of multiple pregnancy'. Cerebral Palsies: Epidemiology and Causal Pathways. London: MacKeith Press; 2000. pp. 109–124, Chapter 10.

[78] Livinec F, Ancel PY, Marret S, et al. The risk of mortality or cerebral palsy in twins: a collaborative population-based study. Pediatr Res 2002;52:671–681.

[79] Little S, Ratcliffe J, Caughey A. Cost of transferring one through five embryos per in vitro fertilization cycle from various payor perspectives. Obstet Gynecol 2006;108(3): 593–601.

[80] Clausson B, Gardosi J, Francis A, Cnattingius S. Perinatal outcome in SGA births defined by customized versus population-based birthweight standards. BJOG 2001;108(8):830–834.

[81] Jensen A, Klonne HJ, Detmer A, Carter AM. Catecholamine and serotonin concentrations in fetal guinea-pig brain: relation to regional cerebral blood flow and oxygen delivery in the growth-restricted fetus. Reprod Fertil Dev 1996;8(3):355–364.

[82] Rees S, Mallard C, Breen S, et al. Fetal brain injury following prolonged hypoxemia and placental insufficiency: a review. Compar Biochem Physiol A. Mol Integr Physiol 1998;119(3):653–660.

[83] Scherjon SA, Oosting H, Smolders-DeHaas H, et al. Neurodevelopmental outcome at three years of age after fetal 'brain-sparing'. Early Hum Dev 1998; 52(1):67–79.

[84] Uvebrant P, Hagberg G. Intrauterine growth in children with cerebral palsy. Acta Paediatr 1992;81(5):407–412.

[85] Ridker PM, Miletich JP, Hennekens C, Buring JE. Ethnic distribution of factor V Leiden in 4047 men and women, implications for venous thromboembolism screening. JAMA 1997;277:1305–1307.

[86] Thorarensen O, Ryan S, Hunter J, Younkin DP. Factor V Leiden mutation: an unrecognized cause of hemiplegic cerebral palsy, neonatal stroke and placental thrombosis. Ann Neurol 1997;42:372–375.

[87] Johnston M, Hagberg H. Sex and the pathogenesis of cerebral palsy. Dev Med Child Neurol 2007;49(1):74–78.

[88] Jacobsson B, Ahlin K, Francis A, et al. Cerebral palsy and restricted growth status at birth: population-based case-control study. BJOG 2008;115(10):1250–1255.

[89] Glinianaia S, Jarvis S, Topp M, et al. Intrauterine growth and cerebral palsy in twins: a European multicenter study. Twin Res Hum Genet 2006;9(3):460–466.

[90] Nelson K. Thrombophilias, perinatal stroke, and cerebral palsy. Clin Obstet Gynecol 2006;49(4):875–884.

[91] Gibson C, MacLennan A, Hague W, et al. Associations between inherited thrombophilias, gestational age, and cerebral palsy. Am J Obstet Gynecol 2005;193(4):1437.

[92] Hong T, Paneth N. Maternal and infant thyroid disorders and cerebral palsy. Semin Perinatol 2008;32(6):438–445.

[93] Garne E, Dolk H, Krageloh-Mann I, et al. Cerebral palsy and congenital malformations. Eur J Paediatr Neurol 2008;12:82–88.

[94] Blair E, Al Asedy F, Badawi N, et al. Is cerebral palsy associated with birth defects other than cerebral defects? Dev Med Child Neurol 2007;49(4):252–258.

[95] Nelson KB. Causative factors in cerebral palsy. Clin Obstet Gynecol 2008;51(4):749–762.

[96] World Health Organization: World Health Report 1998: Life in the twenty first century: a vision for all. Geneva. World Health Organization; 1998.

[97] Powell TG, Pharoah POD, Cooke RWI, Rosenbloom L. Cerebral palsy in low-birth-weight infants. I. Spastic hemiplegia: associations with intrapartum stress. Dev Med Child Neurol 1988;30:11–18.

[98] Hagberg B, Hagberg G, Beckung E, Uvebrant P. Changing panorama of cerebral palsy in Sweden. VIII. Prevalence and origin in the birth year period 1991–94. Acta Paediatr 2001;90(3):271–277.

[99] Blair E, Stanley FJ. Intrapartum asphyxia: a rare cause of cerebral palsy. J Pediatr 1988;112(4):515–519.

[100] Blair E, deGroot J. Prediction or causation: the nature of the association between maternal pre-eclampsia and cerebral palsy. Dev Med Child Neurol 2008;50:32.

[101] Scher A, Petterson B, Blair E, et al. The risk of mortality or cerebral palsy in twins: a collaborative population-based study. Pediatr Res 2002;52:671–681.

[102] Muraskas J, DeGregoris L, Rusciolelli C, Sajous C. Preterm birth of extremely low birth weight infants. In: Morrison J (Ed). Preterm Birth-Mother and Child 2012, pp. 263–274. Rijeka: InTech Open Access Publisher. Available from: http://www.intechopen.com/books/preterm-birth-mother-and-child/preterm-birth-of-extremely-low-birth-weight infants; DOI: 10.5772/32802.

[103] Littenberg B, MacLean C. Passive consent for clinical research in the age of HIPAA. J Gen Intern Med 2006;21(3):207–211.

[104] Cans C, De-la-Cruz J, Mermet MA. Epidemiology of cerebral palsy. Paediatr Child Health 2008;18(9):393–398.

[105] Jacobsson B, Hagberg G, Hagberg B, et al. Cerebral palsy in preterm infants: a population-based casecontrol study of antenatal and intrapartal risk factors. Acta Paediatr 2002;91(8):946–951.

[106] Sanchez PJ. Perinatal infections and brain injury: current treatment options. Clin Perinatol 2002; 29(4):799–826.

[107] Walstab J, Bell R, Reddihough D, Brennecke S, Bessell C, Beischer N. Antenatal and intrapartum antecedents of cerebral palsy a case-control study. Aust NZ J Obstetr Gynaecol 2002;42:138–146.

[108] Nelson KB, Grether JK. Potentially asphyxiating conditions and spastic cerebral palsy in infants of normal birth weight. Am J Obstetr Gynecol 1998;179:507–513.

[109] Laisram N, Srivastava VK, Srivastava RK. Cerebral palsy—an etiological study. Indian J Pediatr 1992; 59:723–728.

[110] Stanley F, Blair E, Alberman E. Post neonatally acquired cerebral palsy: incidence and antecedents. Cerebral Palsies: Epidemiology and Causal Pathways. London: MacKeith Press; 2000. pp. 124–137, Chapter 11.

[111] Pharoah P, Cooke T, Rosenbloom L. Acquired cerebral palsy. Arch Dis Child. 1989;64:1013–1016.

[112] Kerem Günel M, Türker D, Ozal C, Kaya Kara O. Physical management of children with cerebral palsy. In: Emira Svraka (Ed). Cerebral Palsy-Challenges for the Future 2014. pp. 29–73. Rijeka: Available from: http://www.intechopen.com/books/cerebral-palsy-challenges-for-the-future/physical-management-of-children-with-cerebral-palsy; DOI: 10.5772/57505

Section 2

Evaluation

Chapter 2

Assessments and Outcome Measures of Cerebral Palsy

Ayşe Numanoğlu Akbaş

Additional information is available at the end of the chapter

http://dx.doi.org/ 10.5772/64254

Abstract

In cerebral palsy (CP), numerous primary problems are observed including muscle tone problems, muscle weakness, insufficient selective motor control, postural control, and balance problems. In the persistence of these problems for a long period, secondary problems including torsional deformities, joint contractures, scoliosis, and hip dysplasia can occur in time, and strategies formed by children to cope with these problems make up the tertiary problems. Hence, the most accurate and brief assessment of all of these problems mentioned above is crucial to determine an effective and precise physiotherapy program. In the assessment of children with CP, it is very important to receive a detailed story consisting of the birth story, to question underlying medical situations and to carry out physical assessment. In clinics, gross motor function, muscle tone, muscle length, muscle strength, and joint range of motion assessments are the most preferred ones.

Keywords: cerebral palsy, assessment, measurement, evaluation, physiotherapy

1. Introduction

Multidimensional assessment in cerebral palsy (CP) is very important for the determination of the fundamental problems of children, to select the most appropriate therapy approaches for these problems and to reveal the changes occurring during time with the therapy. The assessment should provide information on the primary, secondary, and tertiary problems, functional capacity of the children, and the expectations of the children and families. Although various scales and tests prepared for children with CP can be used, observation, photographs, video records, or computer-supported complicated assessment methods can be used as well.

While selecting the outcome measures, psychometric properties should be considered; however, there is no clear information about how the outcome measures will be selected to reveal the function and health of children ideally [1]. In the selection of the assessment methods, it may be beneficial to consider the dimensions of the International Classification of Functioning, Disability and Health Child and Youth Version (ICF-CY) [2], which is a classification system established by World Health Organization (WHO). When considered in the ICF-CY framework, there are instruments assessing body structures and functions such as problems of muscle tone, muscle strength, and selective motor control; instruments assessing activities and participation such as activities of daily life (ADL) and quality of life; and instruments assessing environmental factors such as impact of the family or the environment. Among these tools, the mostly required ones should be determined for the children. This way, a general opinion can be gathered about the children without much detail. Furthermore, the concerned physicians can examine ultrasound, magnetic resonance (MR), or radiographs as a part of neurologic or orthopedic examination and their results can be combined with the physiotherapy assessments. All of these assessments are crucial not only for establishing a physiotherapy program or to determine the efficiency of the program but also for clarifying the surgical or medical interventions that need to be carried out for the children.

In this chapter, the assessment methods most frequently used by physiotherapists for children with CP are discussed.

2. History and observation

Detailed information should be received from the family or caretakers in all issues related to the children including family history, prenatal, natal and postnatal period, chronologic and corrected age, other accompanying problems, developmental story, adaptive equipment used, therapy approaches applied, medication taken, and educational status of the family [3, 4].

Observational analysis is crucial to determine children's functional skills, spontaneous motions and motion strategies, and the underlying fundamental problems. Thus, it can be decided in which field detailed assessment needs to be carried out. Observational analysis prepared by a specialized physiotherapist completes the standardized tests. During observational analysis, children must be in a setting they can be with their family, and they can feel comfortable and safe. There should be various toys and materials in the setting to reveal the children's capacity and to draw their attention. The assessment room should not be crowded and noisy [3]. Observations provide a general idea to physiotherapists about the general state of the children, quality of movements, capacity and motor strategies developed by the children, protective reactions, and upper and lower extremity functions. Video recordings during observation are rather beneficial as well.

3. Assessment of reflexes and reactions

Observation of reflexes is important to illustrate the severity of the influence in the nervous system, and observation of balance and protective reactions is important to support motor

http://dx.doi.org/ 10.5772/64254

developmental process. When these assessments are carried out, the corrected age of the children should be considered. It is known that primitive reflexes continue insistently or disappear later than normal or never occur in children with CP [5]. It can be observed that symmetric tonic and asymmetric tonic neck reflexes still continue in adolescent stage in a case diagnosed with dyskinetic-type CP. Insistence of these reflexes can complicate the therapy. It may be necessary to make various adaptations in the treatment program when the primitive reflexes continue in advanced ages. For example, in a case whose asymmetric tonic neck reflexes continues, orientation of the head and extremities in the midline may be the fundamental target of the therapy. At the same time, the assessment of protective reactions is important for determining a treatment program.

4. Assessment of functional level and motor development

Although CP is a nonprogressive central nervous system problem, emerging physical impairment and functional limitations change with the therapy approaches applied to the children during growth and with the effect of the environmental conditions. It is crucial to assess motor development, functional skills, and activity limitations for determining the current state of the children, and there are frequently used test batteries for this purpose. Gross Motor Function Measurement (GMFM) [6] is a standardized measurement instrument frequently used to measure the change in gross motor function. This tool consists of five different dimensions, and all skills of the children during supine/prone position, sitting, crawling, standing up, and walking are assessed in detail. GMFM, with versions consisting of 88 items and 66 items, is accepted worldwide. Items 48 and 50 from GMFM 88 version are shown in **Figures 1** and **2**.

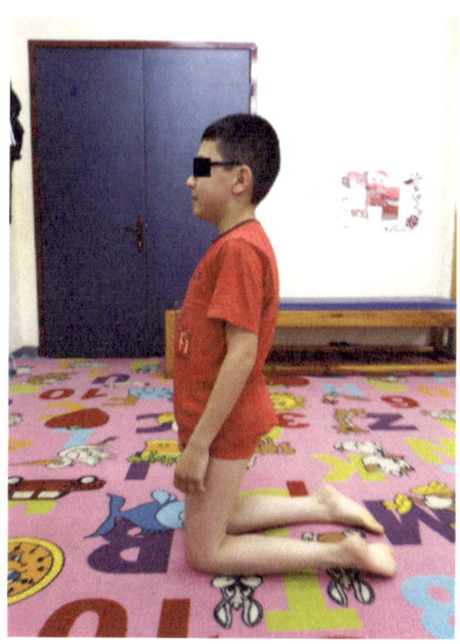

Figure 1. GMFM-88, Item 48.

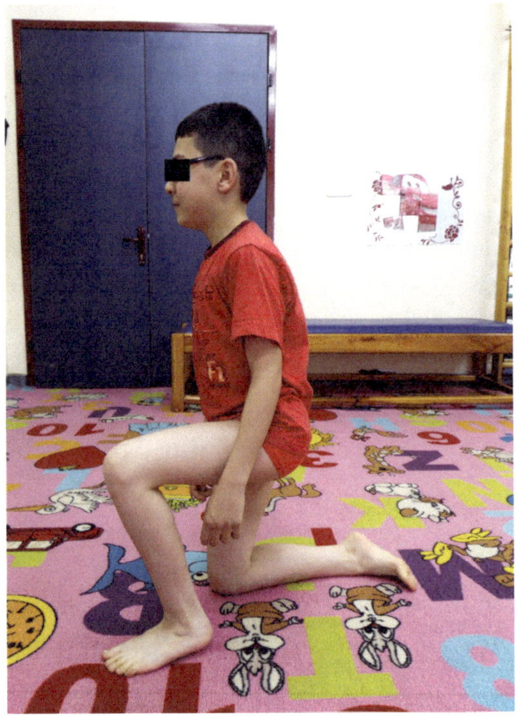

Figure 2. GMFM-88, Item 50.

Gross Motor Function Classification System [7] is the most frequently used classification system interdisciplinary and intradisciplinary to define motor level in children with CP. This classification system categorizes the functional skills of children during their daily life under five levels. In addition, for assessing functional level and motor development various scales are used as well including *Activities Scale for Kids [8], Child Health Questionnaire [9], Gillette Functional Assessment Questionnaire [10], Functional Mobility Scale [11], Pediatric Evaluation of Disability Inventory [12], Pediatric Outcomes Data Collection Instrument [13], and Functional Independence Measure for Children [14].*

5. Assessment of muscle tone

Spastic type is the most common one among CP types. Therefore, spasticity is the major problem encountered most frequently by pediatric physiotherapists. Spasticity makes the voluntary and selective motor control more difficult, increases energy consumption, and causes the formation of secondary musculoskeletal system problems observed in CP [15]. Various physiotherapy methods can be effective in mild tone problems; however, medical or surgical interventions are needed for severe increase in tone persisting for a long time. In this context, it is crucial to determine the changes occurred in muscle tone.

The most affected muscles from spasticity in children with CP are gastroc-soleus, hamstrings, rectus femoris, hip adductors and psoas in lower extremities, and shoulder external rotators, elbow, wrist and finger flexors, and forearm pronators in upper extremities [16].

There are various clinical scales, biomechanical assessment tools, and neurophysiologic assessment methods to assess spasticity; however, there is no consensus about the best assessment. The most frequently used clinical scales are *Ashworth/Modified Ashworth (MAS) and Tardieu/Modified Tardieu (MTS)* scales. MTS grades muscle spasticity in three different velocities and goniometric measurements also included for all velocities [17, 18]. According to a study by Numanoğlu et al. [19], the administration of MAS is easier and takes less time than MTS, but MTS gives valuable information about muscle length and dynamic contracture and has better intraobserver reliability [19]. Assessment of knee flexor muscle spasticity with MTS is shown in **Figure 3**.

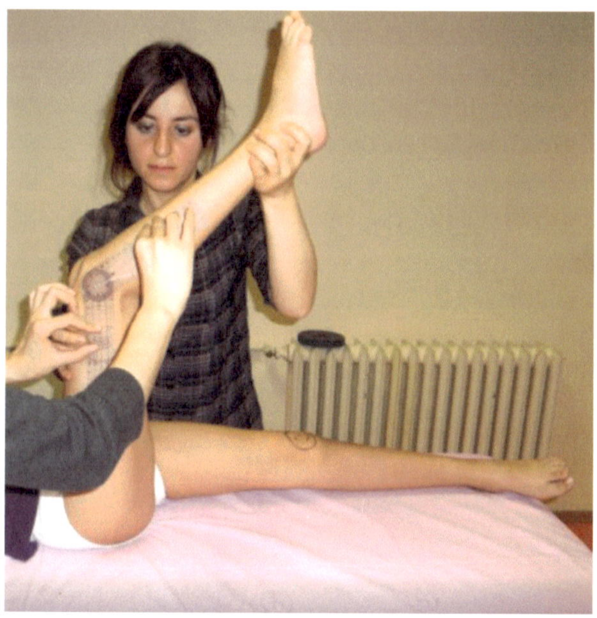

Figure 3. Assessment of knee flexor spasticity with MTS.

In addition to these, there are scales such as *Spasticity Grading, Modified Composite Spasticity Index, Duncan Ely Test, New York University Tone Scale, and the Hypertonia Assessment Tool* [20–22].

Myotonometer, sensors, Wartenberg Pendulum Test, dynamometer, goniometric measurement, and robot-supported assessment instruments are used as biomechanical assessment tools [21, 23–27]. In the neurophysiologic assessment of spasticity, Hoffman H reflex occurring with low-threshold electric stimulation, tendon reflex occurring with tendon tap, and M-wave generated by high-intensity stimulation of peripheral nerve are used. However, overlapping of the values of healthy muscles with those of spastic muscles decreases the diagnostic value of these measurements. Furthermore, electromyography methods are also used in spasticity assessment [21, 28–30].

In the long term spasticity; intrinsic structure of the muscles changes and this leads to muscle stiffness. In a study, an increase in the extracellular matrix collagen density of muscle fiber bundle in spastic hamstrings was reported to be the reason for an increased passive stiffness of muscle, and indicated that this situation can develop even before 3 years of age in children with CP [31–33]. From this perspective, it is important to assess not only neural mechanisms of hypertonus but also nonneural mechanism. In recent years, elastography is benefited in the assessment of muscle stiffness in children with CP [34, 35].

In addition to tone increase in children with CP, hypotonia and muscle fluctuations are observed as well. There are tools to assess dystonia such as *the Burke-Fahn-Marsden Rating Scale [36]* and *Unified Dystonia Rating Scale* [37]. There is no tool used routinely by the clinicians to assess hypotonia; it is generally categorized as mild, moderate, and severe.

6. Assessment of muscle strength

One of the primary problems observed in CP is muscle weakness. This situation occurs due to reasons including central nervous system impairment, inactivation, learned nonuse, and inadequate selective motor control. Muscle weakness can be observed in all subtypes of CP, and it is seen that muscular forces of children with CP are less than those of their peers who developed typically. Moreover, children with CP have slower sequential force generation in force application and have influenced motor planning [38, 39].

Many publications show that strength trainings improve functional capacity without causing any problems in children with CP [40, 41]. In this respect, assessment of muscular force is significant.

Muscular force can be assessed as isometric, isotonic, and isokinetic. For muscle strength assessment, the patients should cooperate with the assessor and the target muscle group must contract maximum; however, it could become difficult due to increased co-contractions in agonist-antagonists and due to cognitive limitations [42]. In the assessment of muscular force, manual muscle testing, testing with handheld dynamometer, and isokinetic dynamometer or the measurement of maximum repetition of functional exercises are used frequently [43].

Usage of handheld dynamometers is suggested in the assessment of upper extremity and lower extremity isometric muscular force and grasping in children with CP [43–46]. A systematic review about this issue suggested that Jamar dynamometer can be used to measure grasping force and handheld dynamometer can be used to measure the force of other upper extremity muscles. It is also reported that manual muscle testing can be used to measure the total upper extremity force or hand wrist force in children who have very limited muscular force [47].

7. Assessment of musculoskeletal system deformities

Children with CP are prone to develop musculoskeletal system deformities. In addition to the major problems generated by central nervous system lesion in CP, secondary problems also exist. The development of musculoskeletal system in children with CP can be affected negatively due to the reasons including muscle weakness, postural problems, and muscle tone problems [50]. Musculoskeletal system should be assessed in detail to detect and to prevent from deformities at an early stage. For this purpose, various measurements should be made such as the measurement of muscular force, range of motion, extremity length, and muscle length.

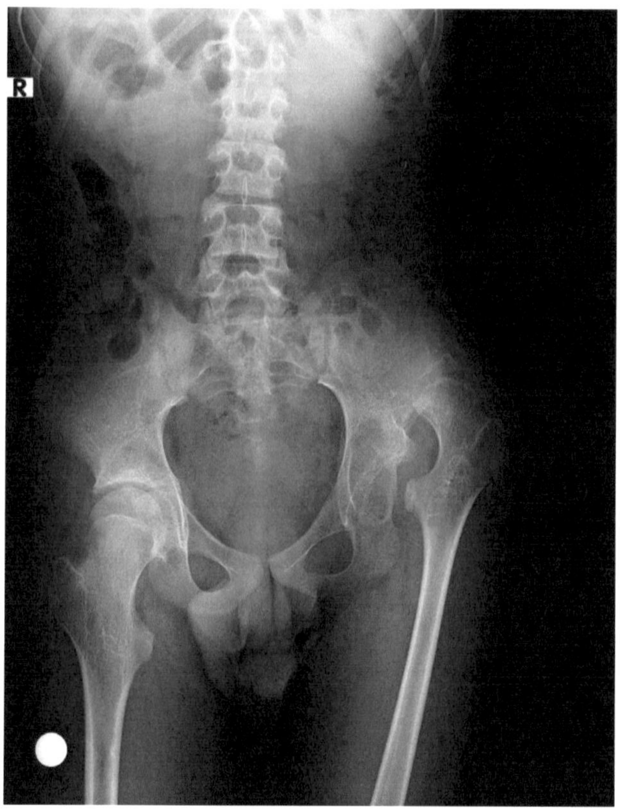

Figure 4. X-ray of a child with quadriparetic CP, age 13, GMFCS Level 5.

Numerous problems concerned with hips can occur in individuals with CP related to aging. Many children with CP are born with a healthy hip; however, scores of problems cause insufficiencies in femur and acetabulum development. These problems are physical inactivity, severe mental retardation, flexion and adduction contractures, pelvic obliquity, sitting in "W" position, excessive tone increase in hip flexor, adductor, and internal rotator muscles, muscular imbalance, and insufficiency in weight bearing [48–50]. Coxavalga, increased femoral anteversion, and acetabular dysplasia are the major problems of hip. Hip subluxation rate in CP is reported to be 75% [51, 52]. Walking ability is the key point in the development of hip problems. Dynamic compressive forces generated during walking are required for the development of the required depth in acetabulum [53]. Hemiparetic and diparetic children, who could walk independently at the age of 30 months, have the lowest risk for hip dislocation [54]. Hip subluxation was reported to be 11% in ambulatory children and 57% in nonambulatory children [49]. Deterioration of motor level affects hip development directly; it was reported that there was 90% hip displacement in children at GMFCS level V [55]. In **Figure 4**, hip X-ray of a 13-year-old child with quadriparetic CP, who was classified in GMFCS level 5, is shown.

Hip surveillance is important for the determination of hip dislocation. Routine radiographic hip assessment is one of the most significant parts of hip follow-up. It was reported that imaging as a part of orthopedic assessment should be carried out at 12–18 months and should be repeated every 6 months [56]. Reimer's Migration Percentage and acetabular index are assessments suggested for radiologic hip monitoring [54]. Children whose Reimer's Migration Percentage is greater than 33% or whose acetabular index is greater than 30% are at risk and they should be monitored closely [48, 54, 57]. For hip surveillance, the hip abduction range of motion at flexion and extension position, presence of contractures, pelvic obliquity, femoral anteversion angle, and spinal deformities should also be assessed [49].

8. Assessment of physical fitness

Due to physical impairments, individuals with CP have more reduced physical fitness in comparison to their peers who develop typically. Tone disorders, muscle weakness, emotional problems, and unfavorable environmental conditions push individuals with CP to move much less in comparison to their peers during the day and to develop sedentary lifestyle [58]. These risks increase in children who are affected bilaterally or have low GMFCS level. In a study conducted on this matter, it was reported that individuals with CP engage in physical activities 13–53% less in comparison to their peers who developed typically and the time spent sedentarily is twofolds higher than that suggested normally [59]. As the age advances, this situation becomes more serious due to the occurrence of musculoskeletal system deformities and the increase of body weight. Because of the abovementioned reasons, children with CP may face many undesired health conditions such as metabolic dysfunction, cardiovascular illness, and decrease in bone mineral density. There are various measurement methods used to assess physical activity. Maintaining an activity journal may help the assessment. Many surveys such as *Activity Scales for Kids [60], Physical Activity Questionnaire for Adolescents [61], Children's Assessment of Participation and Enjoyment [62], Canada Fitness Survey [63], and the Early Activity Scale for Endurance [64]* are benefited for this purpose [65, 66].

General physical endurance can be assessed by a *6-Min Walk Test* [67, 68]. In addition to the surveys, equipment such as step counters, heart rate meters, and accelerometers can be used or more complicated assessment methods such as The Doubly Labelled Water Technique can be applied [69, 70].

http://dx.doi.org/10.5772/64254

9. Assessment of gait

Ensuring independent locomotion is one of the basic goals of many physiotherapists and families of children with CP. Children with unilateral CP almost always develop independent locomotion; however, a part of children with bilateral CP walk independently, some of them walk with aids, and some cannot achieve this function during their lifetime. Numerous gait problems such as equinus, crouch gait, jump gait, and scissoring gait are observed in children with CP who can walk independently.

Gait assessment can be used as an outcome measure to determine the reason of the problem in children and to determine the effects of the interventions [71].

Gait assessment in children with CP can be made by observational gait scale-combined video records, time-distance characteristics, and instrumented gait analyses. Instrumented gait analyses made by measuring electromyography activity, three-dimensional joint kinetic, and kinematic values in laboratory setting present an objective assessment of the patients; however, they are not appropriate for routine clinical purposes. These systems require trained personnel, appropriate setting and the evaluation and interpretation of the results lasts for 3–6 h. In this context, observational gait assessment emerges as an important and useful tool for clinicians. Simple gait scales can be used to determine the quantity of the changes in gait pattern, and deviations from normal gait in the stance and swing phases. In these assessments, clinicians record the walking pattern by video and evaluate walking abnormalities in different joints and planes according to the existing scales. Furthermore, there are computer-supported video analysis programs to be used for this purpose. Among the observational gait assessment tools, there are *Gillette Functional Assessment Questionnaire [10], Physician Rating Scale [72], Observational Gait Scale [73], Visual Gait Score, Salford Gait Tool, Edinburgh Visual Gait Scale [74], Observational Gait Analysis, and Visual Gait Assessment Scale* [71, 75]. According to Günel et al., GMFM's gait domain can also be used as a gait assessment [76]. Among these gait scales, *Edinburgh Visual Gait Scale* is suggested because it consists of information in each of the three planes for foot, knee, hip, pelvis, and trunk for both stance and swing phases and have good reliability and concurrent validity. It is reported that any of these scales is not equivalent to instrumented gait analyses [71].

10. Assessment of balance

Muscle tone impairments and abnormal postural control in children with CP affect balance capacity negatively. It is known that static and dynamic balance reactions of children with CP are insufficient when compared with their normally developed peers [77]. *Pediatric Reach Test [78], Pediatric Balance Scale [79], Timed Up and Go Test [80], Pediatric Clinical Test of Sensory Interaction for Balance [81], Heel-to-Toe Stand, Timed One-Leg Stance, and Timed Up and Down Stairs* are frequently used balance assessments in children with CP. Special equipment such as *Wii-Fit* and *Biodex Balance System* can be benefited as well [82–84].

11. Assessment of trunk impairment

Problems concerned with the trunk are observed frequently in children with CP and these problems affect both upper and lower extremity functions negatively. There are different methods for assessment of the trunk impairment. Assessment of postural control at the sitting position can be used to determine the weakness of the trunk muscles. Moreover, the affected trunk control leads to insufficient balance and therefore instruments assessing postural control and balance during sitting can be benefited to assess the trunk impairment [85].

In the literature, there are limited number of instruments providing information about postural control during sitting and most of the measurements are developed for adults [86]. Some of the scales that could be used to assess trunk impairment in children with CP are listed below:

- *Spinal Alignment and Range-of-Motion Measure* assessing spinal alignment and range of motion [87].
- *Segmental Assessment of Trunk Control* assessing static, active, and reactive sitting balance and control level [88].
- *Seated Postural Control Measure* assessing sitting function and alignment [89].
- *Trunk Control Measurement Scale (TCMS)* assessing static and dynamic sitting balance and dynamic reaching [90].
- *Level of Sitting Scale* classifying sitting ability [91].
- *Assessment & Coding of Postural and Behavioral Observations* assessing head control during sitting, grasping, reaching, eating, and drinking activities [92].
- *Sitting Assessment for Children with Neuromotor Dysfunction* assessing static and dynamic postural control during sitting [93].
- *Seated Posture Control Measurement* assessing postural alignment [94].
- *Sitting Assessment Scale* assessing sitting posture and control with video records [95].
- *Chailey Levels of Ability* assessing sitting, reaching, and standing ability [96].
- *Trunk Impairment Scale* assessing static and dynamic sitting balance of trunk coordination [97, 98].

Furthermore, scales such as *Pediatric Balance Scale, Pediatric Reach Test, Modified Posture Assessment Scale, and Gross Motor Function Measurement* provides information about the trunk although they do not assess trunk impairment directly [78, 84, 86, 99].

Among the scales indicated above, Trunk Control Measurement Scale (TCMS) [90] can be preferred because it has good inter-rater reliability, does not require equipment other than simple materials such as a measuring tape and a ruler, does not require researcher training, and can be used easily in clinical setting. Item 8 of TCMS is shown in **Figures 5** and **6** [84, 86, 100].

http://dx.doi.org/ 10.5772/64254

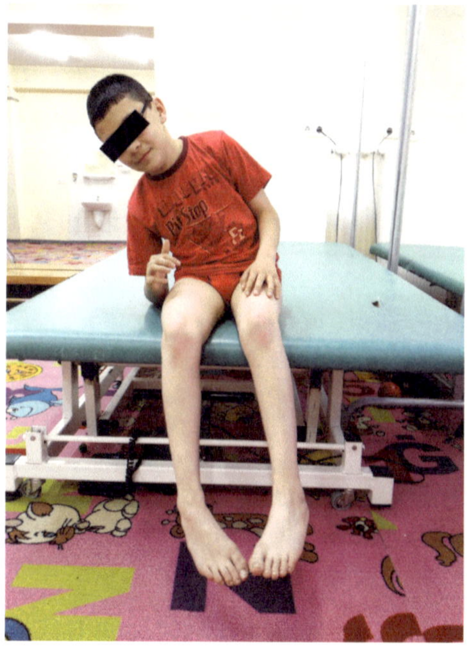

Figure 5. TCMS, Item 8.

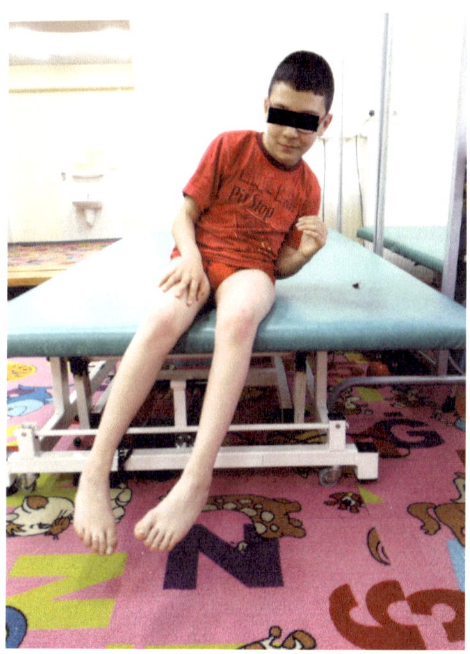

Figure 6. TCMS, Item 8.

12. Assessment of health-related quality of life

Although motor function problems are the major problems in children with CP, with the accompanying sensory, cognitive, and mental problems, activities of daily life and functional independence of the children are influenced as well. Not only children but those of the individuals taking care of them are also affected negatively. It was reported that children with CP experience emotional and behavioral problems fourfolds more than their peers. Quality of life should be self-reported by the person if possible due to its personal nature. However, this may not be possible in children with CP who have severe cognitive impairment; therefore, surveys assessing quality of life need to be answered by family or caretakers [101–103]. Surveys answered by families are used more in children who are under 18 years of age and have difficulty in communication. For children who have no communication problem and can express themselves, child reports should be used. For this purpose, questionnaires such as *Pediatric Outcomes Data Collection Instrument and Child Health Questionnaire [13]* are the most used ones. *Child Health Questionnaire-Parent Form 50 [9], Lifestyle Assessment Questionnaire [104], KIDSCREEN [105], Cerebral Palsy Quality of Life-Child, the Caregiver Priorities and Child Health Index of Life with Disabilities [106], the Pediatric Quality-of-life Inventory CP Module [107], and the DISABKIDS CP Module [108]* that are scored by families are used. According to a systematic review, for children with CP who are at school age, Cerebral Palsy Quality of Life-Child Survey is recommended due to its strongest psychometric properties and clinical utility [3, 101, 109–111].

13. Assessment of activities of daily life

Activities of daily life (ADL) are vital tasks of persons in their school, home, and social environment. According to ICF-CY, these activities are included in the Activity and Participation dimension, including activities such as personal care, nutrition, cleaning, etc. Motor, sensory, perception, cognition, communication, and behavioral problems existing in children with CP can affect ADL performance [112]. Children with CP have difficulty in performing activities of daily life and generally need adaptive equipment or family assistance. Therefore, activities of daily life should be assessed and attempts should be made to develop these activities. According to a systematic review, ADL scales that could be used in children with CP at the age of 5–18 are *ABILHAND-Kids [113], Assessment of Motor and Process Skills [114], Children's Hand-use Experience Questionnaire [115], Klein-Bell Activities of Daily Living [116], Functional Independence Measure for Children [14], Pediatric Evaluation of Disability Inventory [12], School Function Assessment, and Vineland Adaptive Behavior Scales [117].* Among these scales, *Pediatric Evaluation of Disability Inventory* was reported to be the best assessment instrument for children at an elementary school age because of its psychometric properties and personal ADL items. *Children's Hand-use Experience Questionnaire, Vineland Adaptive Behavior Scale, and Functional Independence Measure for Children* were reported to be appropriate for adolescent age. *Assessment of Motor and Process Skills* scale was reported to be the best scale assessing ADL in adolescent children with CP regardless of age [112].

http://dx.doi.org/ 10.5772/64254

14. Assessments of upper extremity

The upper extremity problems are observed in children with unilateral or bilateral CP but these problems can be more important for the children with unilateral involvement because the lower extremity functions are managed in this group more easily.

Motor planning, sensory motor integration, and bimanual coordination problems are observed frequently in the upper extremities *[118]. Manual Ability Classification System (MACS) [119]* classifying the upper extremity function at five levels is used frequently. This system examines the bilateral skills of the extremities during daily life activities. *Assisting Hand Assessment* scale [120] assesses the use of the affected extremity during bilateral activities. Many different scales such as *Melbourne Assessment of Unilateral Upper Limb Function [121], Jebsen Taylor Hand Function Test [122], Zancolli Hand Deformity Classification, Shriners Hospital Upper Extremity Evaluation [123], Upper Extremity Rating Scale, ABILHAND-Kids Questionnaire [113], Bimanual Fine Motor Function, the Quality of Upper Extremity Skills Test [124], and the Canadian Occupational Performance Measure [125]* are used to assess the upper extremity function in children with CP [126]. Two items from *the Quality of Upper Extremity Skills Test* are shown in **Figures 7** and **8**. Also, musculoskeletal evaluation methods, which are mentioned above, can be specified for upper extremities.

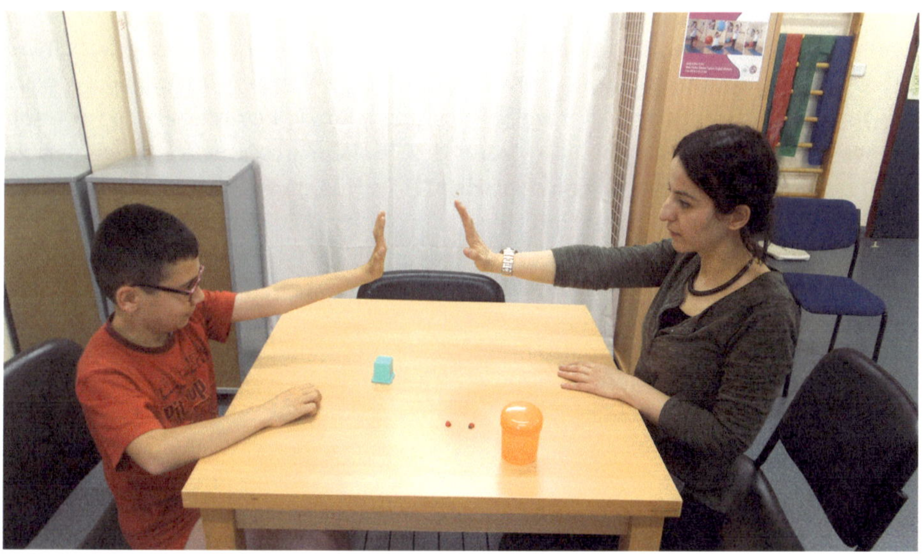

Figure 7. An item from *The Quality of Upper Extremity Skills Test.*

A systematic review reported that any of the scales listed above did not reveal all ICF dimensions in detail on their own and different assessment methods should be combined to assess the upper extremity performance and function in children with CP [127].

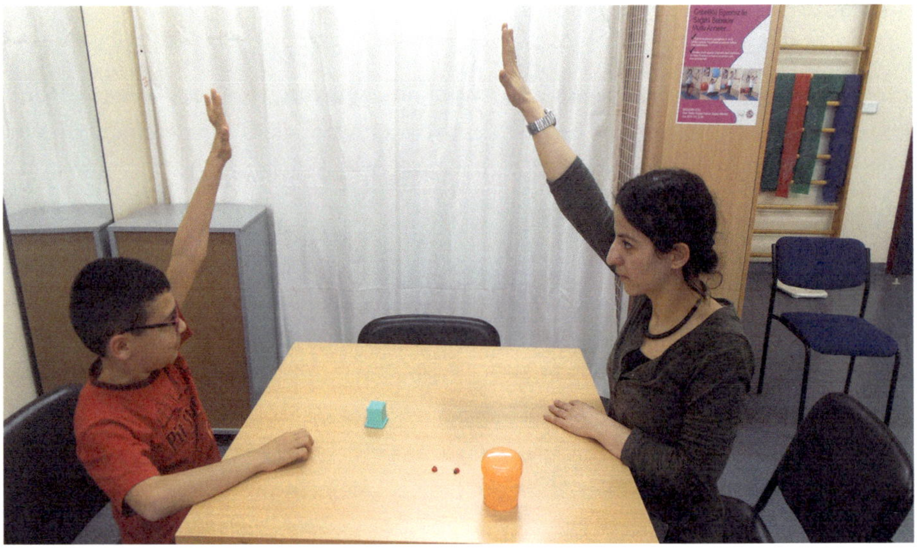

Figure 8. An item from *The Quality of Upper Extremity Skills Test.*

15. Infant assessment

Today, the number of preterm and low birth weight infants is increasing gradually. These infants can present motor impairment findings ranging from developmental coordination disorder to CP in the later stages of development [128]. It may be necessary to wait until 2–3 years of age to diagnose with CP in many countries. In a study conducted in Denmark, it was reported that although CP diagnosis was made at month 11 on an average, the children were not recorded in CP registry system until 4–6 years old for finalizing that the situation is not progressive [129].

However, prior to diagnosis, various assessments should be carried out and motor development should be monitored in especially risky groups. It is suggested that age-appropriate neuromotor assessments of infants with low birth weight and premature infants are made during the first year of life [130]. These assessments are crucial to ensure the differentiation of the infants with motor dysfunction and typically developing, to predict which infants will have motor influence in the future by considering their current performance and to determine the changes occurring in time [131]. Therapy approaches give the best results at this stage when brain development continues rapidly. In this context, infant neuromotor assessments are made to determine infants with motor impairment and to start the early intervention program promptly.

The commonly used assessment instruments for this purpose were reported as *Alberta Infant Motor Scale (AIMS) [132], Bayley Scale of Infant and Toddler Development [133], Peabody Developmental Motor Scales [134], Denver Developmental Screening Test [135], Prechtl's Assessment of*

http://dx.doi.org/ 10.5772/64254

General Movements (GMs) [136], Motion Assessment of Infants, Test of Infant Motor Performance (TIMP) [137], Infant Motor Profile [138], and the Neurological Sensory Motor Developmental Assessment (NSMDA) [139] [5, 131].

Among these assessment methods, some of them such as GMs assess spontaneous movements of infants without any handling and some scales assess both spontaneous behavior and motor behavior occurring with minimal handling. Only TIMP and GMs among the abovementioned tests are appropriate to be used before the term stage. In a systematic review, it was reported that GMs have the best predictive validity for CP during the early infancy stage and AIMS and NSMDA are the best scales for motor development prediction in the later months. The authors of this review suggest that more than one scale should be used in infants. They discuss that the utilization of GMS and TIMP in the preterm phase and their use along with AIMS and NDSMA will give best results in terms of predictive, discriminative, and evaluative assessments. Better results can be obtained with the repetition of the assessments in infants in certain intervals [131].

16. Other assessment methods

In addition to all of these assessments discussed above, it may be necessary to assess other accompanying problems as well. Sleep quality in children with CP can be assessed with *Children's Sleep Habits Questionnaire [140]*, global mental functions can be assessed with *Leiter International Performance Scale [141]*, global psychosocial functions with *Self-perception Profile for Children and Self-perception Profile for Adolescents [142]*, attention functions with *Behaviour Rating Inventory of Executive Function [143]*, communication skills with *Preschool Language Scale [144] and Communication Function Classification System [145]*, voluntary motion control with *Selective Control Assessment of the Lower Extremity [146]*, eating and drinking function with *Eating and Drinking Ability Classification System [147]*, and saliva control can be assessed with *Drool Severity Score* [145].

Pain is one of the frequently observed problems in especially advanced ages in children with CP; scores of factors can be discussed causing pain such as contractures, hip dislocation, patella alta, equines deformity, dysphagia, gastroesophageal reflux, gastrointestinal tube feeding, and constipation. Also, pain can develop originating from the used adaptive equipment and orthosis or as a result of physiotherapy, serial casting, and surgical interventions. Whereas information about pain can be assessed simply by asking the children and families or can be assessed with scales such as *Non-Communicating Children's Pain Checklist [148] and Pediatric Pain Profile (PPP)* [149]. For children who have communication problems, parent proxy reports can be used. However, monitoring of findings including spontaneous motions, facial expression, breathing pattern, sweating, or blushing also provides opinion about pain.

Children with CP have numerous motor, sensorial, and behavioral problems as discussed in detail above. Moreover, these problems may give different findings along with growth. Application of protective methods is necessary before the generation of many problems. In this sense, assessments are crucial. The current state of children and changes occurred with treatments can be observed in detail when the most appropriate assessment is selected from the assessments discussed above by considering ICF dimensions. Thus, both body structure and functions and activity and participation of children with CP can be improved, and inclusion of them in a society as healthier and happier individuals can be assisted.

Author details

Ayşe Numanoğlu Akbaş

Address all correspondence to: aysenumanoglu@gmail.com

Department of Physical Therapy and Rehabilitation, Abant İzzet Baysal University, Bolu, Turkey

References

[1] Schiariti, V., et al., *Comparing contents of outcome measures in cerebral palsy using the international classification of functioning (ICF-CY): a systematic review*. European Journal of Paediatric Neurology, 2014. 18(1): pp. 1–12.

[2] World Health Organization, International Classification of Functioning, Disability, and Health: Children & Youth Version: ICF-CY. 2007: World Health Organization, Geneva, Switzerland.

[3] Livanelioğlu, A. and Kerem Gunel, M., Physiotherapy of Cerebral Palsy. 2009: Yeni Özbek Press, Ankara Turkey.

[4] Miller, F., Physical Therapy of Cerebral Palsy. 2007. Springer Science+Business Media, New York, USA.

[5] Zafeiriou, D.I., *Primitive reflexes and postural reactions in the neurodevelopmental examination*. Pediatric Neurology, 2004. 31(1): pp. 1–8.

[6] Russell, D.J., et al., Gross Motor Function Measure (GMFM-66 and GMFM-88) User's Manual. 2002: Cambridge University Press., Cambridge, United Kingdom.

[7] Palisano, R., et al., *Development and reliability of a system to classify gross motor function in children with cerebral palsy*. Developmental Medicine & Child Neurology, 1997. 39(4): pp. 214–223.

[8] Plint, A.C., et al., *Activities scale for kids: an analysis of normals*. Journal of Pediatric Orthopaedics, 2003. 23(6): pp. 788–790.

[9] Landgraf, J.M., L. Abetz, and J.E. Ware, *Child Health Questionnaire (CHQ): A User's Manual*. 1996: Boston: Health Institute, New England Medical Center.

[10] Novacheck, T.F., J.L. Stout, and R. Tervo, *Reliability and validity of the Gillette functional assessment questionnaire as an outcome measure in children with walking disabilities*. Journal of Pediatric Orthopaedics, 2000. 20(1): p. 75.

[11] Graham, H.K., et al., *The functional mobility scale (FMS)*. Journal of Pediatric Orthopaedics, 2004. 24(5): pp. 514–520.

[12] Haley, S., et al., Pediatric evaluation of disability inventory. Assessing children's wellbeing: a handbook of measures, 2003. 11: p. 13. Pennsylvania University Press, Pennsylvania, USA.

[13] Lerman, J.A., et al., *The Pediatric Outcomes Data Collection Instrument (PODCI) and functional assessment of patients with unilateral upper extremity deficiencies*. Journal of Pediatric Orthopaedics, 2005. 25(3): pp. 405–407.

[14] Hamilton, B. and C. Granger, *Functional Independence Measure for Children (WeeFIM)*. 1991: Buffalo, NY: Research Foundation of the State University of New York.

[15] Morrell, D.S., J.M. Pearson, and D.D. Sauser, *Progressive bone and joint abnormalities of the spine and lower extremities in cerebral palsy 1*. Radiographics, 2002. 22(2): pp. 257–268.

[16] Klingels, K., et al., *Upper limb impairments and their impact on activity measures in children with unilateral cerebral palsy*. European Journal of Paediatric Neurology, 2012. 16(5): pp. 475–484.

[17] Bohannon, R.W. and M.B. Smith, *Interrater reliability of a modified Ashworth scale of muscle spasticity*. Physical Therapy, 1987. 67(2): pp. 206–207.

[18] Haugh, A., A. Pandyan, and G. Johnson, *A systematic review of the Tardieu Scale for the measurement of spasticity*. Disability and Rehabilitation, 2006. 28(15): pp. 899–907.

[19] Numanoğlu, A., and M. K. Günel. "Intraobserver reliability of modified Ashworth scale and modified Tardieu scale in the assessment of spasticity in children with cerebral palsy." *Acta orthopaedica et traumatologica turcica* (2011) 46.3: pp 196–200.

[20] Scholtes, V.A., et al., *Clinical assessment of spasticity in children with cerebral palsy: a critical* 18 *review of available instruments*. Developmental Medicine & Child Neurology, 2006. 48(1): 19 pp. 64–73.

[21] Flamand, V.H., H. Massé-Alarie, and C. Schneider, *Psychometric evidence of spasticity measurement tools in cerebral palsy children and adolescents: a systematic review*. Journal of Rehabilitation Medicine, 2013. 45(1): pp. 14–23.

[22] Jethwa, A., et al., *Development of the Hypertonia Assessment Tool (HAT): a discriminative tool for hypertonia in children*. Developmental Medicine & Child Neurology, 2010. 52(5): pp. e83–e87.

[23] Leonard, C.T., J.U. Stephens, and S.L. Stroppel, *Assessing the spastic condition of individuals with upper motoneuron involvement: validity of the myotonometer*. Archives of Physical Medicine and Rehabilitation, 2001. 82(10): pp. 1416–1420.

[24] Syczewska, M., M.K. Lebiedowska, and A.D. Pandyan, *Quantifying repeatability of the Wartenberg pendulum test parameters in children with spasticity*. Journal of Neuroscience Methods, 2009. 178(2): pp. 340–344.

[25] Boiteau, M., F. Malouin, and C.L. Richards, *Use of a hand–held dynamometer and a Kin-Com® dynamometer for evaluating spastic hypertonia in children: a reliability study*. Physical Therapy, 1995. 75(9): pp. 796–802.

[26] van den Noort, J.C., V.A. Scholtes, and J. Harlaar, *Evaluation of clinical spasticity assessment in cerebral palsy using inertial sensors*. Gait & Posture, 2009. 30(2): pp. 138–143.

[27] Schmartz, A.C., et al., *Measurement of muscle stiffness using robotic assisted gait orthosis in children with cerebral palsy: a proof of concept*. Disability and Rehabilitation: Assistive Technology, 2011. 6(1): pp. 29–37.

[28] Bar-On, L., et al., Spasticity and its contribution to hypertonia in cerebral palsy. BioMed Research International, 2015. p 1–10

[29] Kohan, A.H., et al., *Comparison of modified Ashworth scale and Hoffmann reflex in study of spasticity*. Acta Medica Iranica, 2010. 48(3): pp. 154–157.

[30] Poon, D.M. and C.W. HUI-CHAN, *Hyperactive stretch reflexes, co-contraction, and muscle weakness in children with cerebral palsy*. Developmental Medicine & Child Neurology, 2009. 51(2): pp. 128–135.

[31] Willerslev-Olsen, M., et al., *Passive muscle properties are altered in children with cerebral palsy before the age of 3 years and are difficult to distinguish clinically from spasticity*. Developmental Medicine & Child Neurology, 2013. 55(7): pp. 617–623.

[32] Barber, L., R. Barrett, and G. Lichtwark, *Passive muscle mechanical properties of the medial gastrocnemius in young adults with spastic cerebral palsy*. Journal of Biomechanics, 2011. 44(13): pp. 2496–2500.

[33] Smith, L.R., et al., *Hamstring contractures in children with spastic cerebral palsy result from a stiffer extracellular matrix and increased in vivo sarcomere length*. The Journal of Physiology, 2011. 589(10): pp. 2625–2639.

[34] Kwon, D.R., G.Y. Park, and J.G. Kwon, *The change of intrinsic stiffness in gastrocnemius after intensive rehabilitation with botulinum toxin A injection in spastic diplegic cerebral palsy*. Annals of Rehabilitation Medicine, 2012. 36(3): pp. 400–403.

[35] Park, G.-Y. and D.R. Kwon, *Sonoelastographic evaluation of medial gastrocnemius muscles intrinsic stiffness after rehabilitation therapy with botulinum toxin a injection in spastic cerebral palsy*. Archives of Physical Medicine and Rehabilitation, 2012. 93(11): pp. 2085–2089.

[36] Krystkowiak, P., et al., *Reliability of the Burke-Fahn-Marsden scale in a multicenter trial for dystonia*. Movement Disorders, 2007. 22(5): pp. 685–689.

[37] Comella, C.L., et al., *Rating scales for dystonia: a multicenter assessment*. Movement Disorders, 2003. 18(3): pp. 303–312.

[38] Smits-Engelsman, B., K. Klingels, and H. Feys, Bimanual force coordination in children with spastic unilateral cerebral palsy. Research in Developmental Disabilities, 2011. 32(5).pp 2011–2019.

[39] Gordon, A.M., J. Charles, and B. Steenbergen, *Fingertip force planning during grasp is disrupted by impaired sensorimotor integration in children with hemiplegic cerebral palsy*. Pediatric Research, 2006. 60(5): pp. 587–591.

[40] Dodd, K.J., N.F. Taylor, and D.L. Damiano, *A systematic review of the effectiveness of strength-training programs for people with cerebral palsy*. Archives of Physical Medicine and Rehabilitation, 2002. 83(8): pp. 1157–1164.

[41] Damiano, D.L. and M.F. Abel, *Functional outcomes of strength training in spastic cerebral palsy*. Archives of Physical Medicine and Rehabilitation, 1998. 79(2): pp. 119–125.

[42] Damiano, D.L., K. Dodd, and N.F. Taylor, *Should we be testing and training muscle strength in cerebral palsy?* Developmental Medicine & Child Neurology, 2002. 44(01): pp. 68–72.

[43] Verschuren, O., et al., *Reliability of hand-held dynamometry and functional strength tests for the lower extremity in children with cerebral palsy*. Disability and Rehabilitation, 2008. 30(18): pp. 1358–1366.

[44] Hwang, A.-W., et al., Reliability of Nicholas hand-held dynamometer of muscle strength measurement in children with cerebral palsy and non-disabled children. *Physiotherapy*, 2002. 27(2): 10 pp. 69–82.

[45] Mulder-Brouwer, A. N., Rameckers, E. A., & Bastiaenen, C. H. (2016). Lower Extremity Handheld Dynamometry Strength Measurement in Children With Cerebral Palsy. *Pediatric Physical Therapy*, 28(2), 136–153.

[46] Willemse, L., et al., *Reliability of isometric lower-extremity muscle strength measurements in children with cerebral palsy: implications for measurement design*. Physical Therapy, 2013. 93(7): pp. 935–941.

[47] Dekkers, K.J., et al., *Upper extremity strength measurement for children with cerebral palsy: a systematic review of available instruments*. Physical Therapy, 2014. 94(5): pp. 609–622.

[48] Yildiz, C. and I. Demirkale, *Hip problems in cerebral palsy: screening, diagnosis and treatment*. Current Opinion in Pediatrics, 2014. 26(1): pp. 85–92.

[49] Chan, G. and F. Miller, *Assessment and treatment of children with cerebral palsy*. Orthopedic Clinics of North America, 2014. 45(3): pp. 313–325.

[50] Tarsuslu, T. and F. Dokuztug, Investigation of the different factors that cause hip problems in spastic quadriparetic cerebral palsy children. Turkish Pediatric Journal, 2008. 51(2): pp. 86.

[51] Hägglund, G., H. Lauge-Pedersen, and P. Wagner, *Characteristics of children with hip displacement in cerebral palsy*. BMC Musculoskeletal Disorders, 2007. 8(1): p. 1.

[52] Morton, R., et al., *Dislocation of the hips in children with bilateral spastic cerebral palsy, 1985–2000*. Developmental Medicine & Child Neurology, 2006. 48(07): pp. 555–558.

[53] Palisano, R. J., Campbell, S. K., & Orlin, M. (2014). *Physical therapy for children*. Elsevier Health Sciences Inc. Missouri, USA pp 183–204.

[54] Gordon, G. and D.E. Simkiss, *A systematic review of the evidence for hip surveillance in children with cerebral palsy*. Journal of Bone & Joint Surgery, British Volume, 2006. 88(11): pp. 1492–1496.

[55] Soo, B., et al., *Hip displacement in cerebral palsy*. The Journal of Bone & Joint Surgery, 2006. 88(1): pp. 121–129.

[56] Spiegel, D.A. and J.M. Flynn, *Evaluation and treatment of hip dysplasia in cerebral palsy*. Orthopedic Clinics of North America, 2006. 37(2): pp. 185–196.

[57] Terjesen, T., *Development of the hip joints in unoperated children with cerebral palsy: a radiographic study of 76 patients*. Acta Orthopaedica, 2006. 77(1): pp. 125–131.

[58] Maher, C.A., et al., *Physical and sedentary activity in adolescents with cerebral palsy*. Developmental Medicine & Child Neurology, 2007. 49(6): pp. 450–457.

[59] Ziegler, K., *Physical Activity and Body Composition in Children with Cerebral Palsy*. 2015: Texas: Texas Christian University Fort Worth.

[60] Young, N.L., et al., *Measurement properties of the activities scale for kids*. Journal of Clinical Epidemiology, 2000. 53(2): pp. 125–137.

[61] Crocker, P., et al., *Measuring general levels of physical activity: preliminary evidence for the Physical Activity Questionnaire for Older Children*. Medicine and Science in Sports and Exercise, 1997. 29(10): pp. 1344–1349.

[62] King, G.A., et al., Children's Assessment of Participation and Enjoyment (CAPE) and Preferences for Activities of Children (PAC). 2000: Pearson Corporate Communications., San Antonio, USA.

[63] Weller, I. and P.N. Corey, *A study of the reliability of the Canada Fitness Survey questionnaire*. Medicine and Science in Sports and Exercise, 1998. 30(10): pp. 1530–1536.

[64] McCoy, S.W., et al., *Development of the early activity scale for endurance for children with cerebral palsy*. Pediatric Physical Therapy, 2012. 24(3): pp. 232–240.

[65] Capio, C.M., et al., *Physical activity measurement instruments for children with cerebral palsy: a systematic review*. Developmental Medicine & Child Neurology, 2010. 52(10): pp. 908–916.

[66] Law, M., et al., *Participation of children with physical disabilities: relationships with diagnosis, physical function, and demographic variables*. Scandinavian Journal of Occupational Therapy, 2004. 11(4): pp. 156–162.

[67] Wright, F.V. and A. Majnemer, *The concept of a toolbox of outcome measures for children with cerebral palsy why, what, and how to use?* Journal of Child Neurology, 2014. 29(8): pp. 1055–1065.

[68] Thompson, P., et al., *Test–retest reliability of the 10-metre fast walk test and 6-minute walk test in ambulatory school-aged children with cerebral palsy.* Developmental Medicine & Child Neurology, 2008. 50(5): pp. 370–376.

[69] Bjornson, K.F., et al., *Ambulatory physical activity performance in youth with cerebral palsy and youth who are developing typically.* Physical Therapy, 2007. 87(3): pp. 248–257.

[70] Mitre, N., et al., *Pedometer accuracy for children: can we recommend them for our obese population?* Pediatrics, 2009. 123(1): pp. e127–e131.

[71] Rathinam, C., et al., *Observational gait assessment tools in paediatrics—a systematic review.* Gait & Posture, 2014. 40(2): pp. 279–285.

[72] Maathuis, K.G., et al., *Gait in children with cerebral palsy: observer reliability of physician rating scale and Edinburgh visual gait analysis interval testing scale.* Journal of Pediatric Orthopaedics, 2005. 25(3): pp. 268–272.

[73] Mackey, A.H., et al., *Reliability and validity of the observational gait scale in children with spastic diplegia.* Developmental Medicine & Child Neurology, 2003. 45(01): pp. 4–11.

[74] Read, H.S., et al., *Edinburgh visual gait score for use in cerebral palsy.* Journal of Pediatric Orthopaedics, 2003. 23(3): pp. 296–301.

[75] Dickens, W.E. and M.F. Smith, *Validation of a visual gait assessment scale for children with hemiplegic cerebral palsy.* Gait & Posture, 2006. 23(1): pp. 78–82.

[76] Günel, M.K., et al., Physical management of children with cerebral palsy. 2014. Intech Press, Rijeka, Croatia.

[77] Gan, S.-M., et al., *Psychometric properties of functional balance assessment in children with cerebral palsy.* Neurorehabilitation and Neural Repair, 2008. 22(6): pp. 745–753.

[78] Bartlett, D. and T. Birmingham, *Validity and reliability of a pediatric reach test.* Pediatric Physical Therapy, 2003. 15(2): pp. 84–92.

[79] Franjoine, M.R., J.S. Gunther, and M.J. Taylor, *Pediatric balance scale: a modified version of the berg balance scale for the school-age child with mild to moderate motor impairment.* Pediatric Physical Therapy, 2003. 15(2): pp. 114–128.

[80] Williams, E.N., et al., *Investigation of the timed 'up & go' test in children.* Developmental Medicine & Child Neurology, 2005. 47(08): pp. 518–524.

[81] Crowe, T.K., et al., *Interrater reliability of the pediatric clinical test of sensory interaction for balance.* Physical & Occupational Therapy in Pediatrics, 1991. 10(4): pp. 1–27.

[82] Goble, D.J., B.L. Cone, and B.W. Fling, *Using the Wii Fit as a tool for balance assessment and neurorehabilitation: the first half decade of "Wii-search"*. Journal of Neuroengineering and Rehabilitation, 2014. 11(1): p. 1.

[83] El-Shamy, S.M. and E.M. Abd El Kafy, *Effect of balance training on postural balance control and risk of fall in children with diplegic cerebral palsy*. Disability and Rehabilitation, 2014. 36(14): pp. 1176–1183.

[84] Saether, R., et al., *Clinical tools to assess balance in children and adults with cerebral palsy: a systematic review*. Developmental Medicine & Child Neurology, 2013. 55(11): pp. 988–999.

[85] Jeong, J., et al., *A reliability of the prototype trunk training system for sitting balance*. Journal of Physical Therapy Science, 2014. 26(11): p. 1745.

[86] Field, D. and R. Livingstone, *Clinical tools that measure sitting posture, seated postural control or functional abilities in children with motor impairments: a systematic review*. Clinical Rehabilitation, 2013: p. 0269215513488122.

[87] Bartlett, D. and B. Purdie, *Testing of the spinal alignment and range of motion measure: a discriminative measure of posture and flexibility for children with cerebral palsy*. Developmental Medicine & Child Neurology, 2005. 47(11): pp. 739–743.

[88] Butler, P., et al., *Refinement, reliability and validity of the segmental assessment of trunk control (SATCo)*. Pediatric Physical Therapy: The Official Publication of the Section on Pediatrics of the American Physical Therapy Association, 2010. 22(3): p. 246.

[89] Fife, S.E., et al., *Development of a clinical measure of postural control for assessment of adaptive seating in children with neuromotor disabilities*. Physical Therapy, 1991. 71(12): pp. 981–993.

[90] Heyrman, L., et al., *A clinical tool to measure trunk control in children with cerebral palsy: the trunk control measurement scale*. Research in Developmental Disabilities, 2011. 32(6): pp. 2624–2635.

[91] Field, D.A. and L.A. Roxborough, *Responsiveness of the seated postural control measure and the level of sitting scale in children with neuromotor disorders*. Disability & Rehabilitation: Assistive Technology, 2011. 6(6): pp. 473–482.

[92] Hulme, J.B., et al., *Behavioral and postural changes observed with use of adaptive seating by clients with multiple handicaps*. Physical Therapy, 1987. 67(7): pp. 1060–1067.

[93] Knox, V., *Evaluation of the sitting assessment test for children with neuromotor dysfunction as a measurement tool in cerebral palsy*. Physiotherapy, 2002. 88(9): pp. 534–541.

[94] McDonald, R. and R. Surtees, *Changes in postural alignment when using kneeblocks for children with severe motor disorders*. Disability & Rehabilitation: Assistive Technology, 2007. 2(5): pp. 287–291.

[95] Myhr, U. and L. Wendt, *Improvement of functional sitting position for children with cerebral palsy*. Developmental Medicine & Child Neurology, 1991. 33(3): pp. 246–256.

[96] Pountney, T.E., et al., *Content and criterion validation of the Chailey levels of ability*. Physiotherapy, 1999. 85(8): pp. 410–416.

[97] Sæther, R. and L. Jørgensen, *Intra-and inter-observer reliability of the Trunk Impairment Scale for children with cerebral palsy*. Research in Developmental Disabilities, 2011. 32(2): pp. 727–739.

[98] Verheyden, G., et al., *The Trunk Impairment Scale: a new tool to measure motor impairment of the trunk after stroke*. Clinical Rehabilitation, 2004. 18(3): pp. 326–334.

[99] Chen, C.-l., et al., *Validity, responsiveness, minimal detectable change, and minimal clinically important change of Pediatric Balance Scale in children with cerebral palsy*. Research in Developmental Disabilities, 2013. 34(3): pp. 916–922.

[100] Bañas, B.B. and E.J.R. Gorgon, *Clinimetric properties of sitting balance measures for children with cerebral palsy: a systematic review*. Physical & Occupational Therapy in Pediatrics, 2014. 34(4): pp. 313–334.

[101] Gilson, K.-M., et al., *Quality of life in children with cerebral palsy implications for practice*. Journal of Child Neurology, 2014. 29(8): pp. 1134–1140.

[102] Glenn, S., et al., *Maternal parenting stress and its correlates in families with a young child with cerebral palsy*. Child: Care, Health and Development, 2009. 35(1): pp. 71–78.

[103] Sigurdardottir, S., et al., *Behavioural and emotional symptoms of preschool children with cerebral palsy: a population-based study*. Developmental Medicine & Child Neurology, 2010. 52(11): pp. 1056–1061.

[104] Mackie, P., E. Jessen, and S. Jarvis, *The lifestyle assessment questionnaire: an instrument to measure the impact of disability on the lives of children with cerebral palsy and their families*. Child: Care, Health and Development, 1998. 24(6): pp. 473–486.

[105] Ravens-Sieberer, U., et al., *KIDSCREEN-52 quality-of-life measure for children and adolescents*. Expert Review of Pharmacoeconomics & Outcomes Research, 2005. 5(3): pp. 353–364.

[106] Narayanan, U., et al., *Caregiver priorities & child health index of life with disabilities: initial development and validation of an outcome measure of health status and well-being in children with severe cerebral palsy*. Developmental Medicine and Child Neurology, 2006. 48: pp. 804–812.

[107] Varni, J.W., M. Seid, and C.A. Rode, *The PedsQL™: measurement model for the pediatric quality of life inventory*. Medical Care, 1999. 37(2): pp. 126–139.

[108] Baars, R.M., et al., *The European DISABKIDS project: development of seven condition-specific modules to measure health related quality of life in children and adolescents*. Health and Quality of Life Outcomes, 2005. 3(1): p. 1.

[109] Schneider, J.W., et al., *Health-related quality of life and functional outcome measures for children with cerebral palsy*. Developmental Medicine & Child Neurology, 2001. 43(09): pp. 601–608.

[110] Waters, E., et al., *Psychometric properties of the quality of life questionnaire for children with CP*. Developmental Medicine & Child Neurology, 2007. 49(1): pp. 49–55.

[111] Carlon, S., et al., *A systematic review of the psychometric properties of Quality of Life measures for school aged children with cerebral palsy*. BMC Pediatrics, 2010. 10(1): p. 1.

[112] James, S., J. Ziviani, and R. Boyd, *A systematic review of activities of daily living measures for children and adolescents with cerebral palsy*. Developmental Medicine & Child Neurology, 2014. 56(3): pp. 233–244.

[113] Arnould, C., et al., *ABILHAND-Kids A measure of manual ability in children with cerebral palsy*. Neurology, 2004. 63(6): pp. 1045–1052.

[114] Fisher, A.G. and K.B. Jones, *Assessment of Motor and Process Skills*. Vol. 375. 1999: Three Star Press Fort Collins, CO.

[115] Sköld, A., et al., *Development and evidence of validity for the Children's Hand-use Experience Questionnaire (CHEQ)*. Developmental Medicine & Child Neurology, 2011. 53(5): pp. 436–442.

[116] Law, M. and P. Usher, *Validation of the Klein-Bell activities of daily living scale for children*. Canadian Journal of Occupational Therapy, 1988. 55(2): pp. 63–68.

[117] Sparrow, S.S., Vineland Adaptive Behavior Scales. 2011: Springer. New York, USA.

[118] Gordon, A.M., Y. Bleyenheuft, and B. Steenbergen, *Pathophysiology of impaired hand function in children with unilateral cerebral palsy*. Developmental Medicine & Child Neurology, 2013. 55(s4): pp. 32–37.

[119] Eliasson, A.-C., et al., *The Manual Ability Classification System (MACS) for children with cerebral palsy: scale development and evidence of validity and reliability*. Developmental Medicine & Child Neurology, 2006. 48(07): pp. 549–554.

[120] Krumlinde-Sundholm, L., et al., *The Assisting Hand Assessment: current evidence of validity, reliability, and responsiveness to change*. Developmental Medicine & Child Neurology, 2007. 49(4): pp. 259–264.

[121] Randall, M., et al., *Reliability of the Melbourne assessment of unilateral upper limb function*. Developmental Medicine & Child Neurology, 2001. 43(11): pp. 761–767.

[122] Lynch, K.B. and M.J. Bridle, *Validity of the Jebsen-Taylor Hand Function Test in predicting activities of daily living*. OTJR, 1989. 9(5): p. 316.

[123] Davids, J.R., et al., *Validation of the Shriners Hospital for Children Upper Extremity Evaluation (SHUEE) for children with hemiplegic cerebral palsy*. Journal of Bone and Joint Surgery. American Volume, 2006. 88(2): pp. 326–333.

[124] DeMatteo, C., et al., *The reliability and validity of the quality of upper extremity skills test.* Physical & Occupational Therapy in Pediatrics, 1993. 13(2): pp. 1–18.

[125] Law, M., et al., *The Canadian occupational performance measure: an outcome measure for occupational therapy.* Canadian Journal of Occupational Therapy, 1990. 57(2): pp. 82–87.

[126] Gilmore, R., L. Sakzewski, and R. Boyd, *Upper limb activity measures for 5-to 16-year-old children with congenital hemiplegia: a systematic review.* Developmental Medicine & Child Neurology, 2010. 52(1): pp. 14–21.

[127] Wagner, L.V. and J.R. Davids, *Assessment tools and classification systems used for the upper extremity in children with cerebral palsy.* Clinical Orthopaedics and Related Research®, 2012. 470(5): pp. 1257–1271.

[128] Bracewell, M. and N. Marlow, *Patterns of motor disability in very preterm children.* Mental Retardation and Developmental Disabilities Research Reviews, 2002. 8(4): pp. 241–248.

[129] Granild-Jensen, J.B., et al., *Predictors for early diagnosis of cerebral palsy from national registry data.* Developmental Medicine & Child Neurology, 2015. 57(10): pp. 931–935.

[130] Wang, C.J., et al., *Quality-of-care indicators for the neurodevelopmental follow-up of very low birth weight children: results of an expert panel process.* Pediatrics, 2006. 117(6): pp. 2080–2092.

[131] Spittle, A.J., L.W. Doyle, and R.N. Boyd, *A systematic review of the clinimetric properties of neuromotor assessments for preterm infants during the first year of life.* Developmental Medicine & Child Neurology, 2008. 50(4): pp. 254–266.

[132] Piper, M.C. and J. Darrah, *Alberta Infant Motor Scale (AIMS).* 1994: Philadelphia: Saunders.

[133] Bayley, N., Bayley Scales of Infant Development: Manual. 1993: Psychological Corporation, San Antonio, USA.

[134] Folio, M.R. and R.R. Fewell, Peabody Developmental Motor Scales: Examiner's Manual. 2000: Pro-ed Press. San Antonio, USA.

[135] Frankenburg, W.K. and J.B. Dodds, *The Denver developmental screening test.* The Journal of Pediatrics, 1967. 71(2): pp. 181–191.

[136] Einspieler, C. and H.F. Prechtl, *Prechtl's assessment of general movements: a diagnostic tool for the functional assessment of the young nervous system.* Mental Retardation and Developmental Disabilities Research Reviews, 2005. 11(1): pp. 61–67.

[137] Campbell, S., et al., *Development of the test of infant motor performance.* Physical Medicine and Rehabilitation Clinics of North America, 1993. 4: pp. 541–541.

[138] Heineman, K.R., A.F. Bos, and M. Hadders-Algra, *The Infant Motor Profile: a standardized and qualitative method to assess motor behaviour in infancy.* Developmental Medicine & Child Neurology, 2008. 50(4): pp. 275–282.

[139] BURNS, Y.R., R.M. ENSBEY, and M.A. NORRIE, *The neuro-sensory motor developmental assessment part 1: development and administration of the test.* Australian Journal of Physiotherapy, 1989. 35(3): pp. 141–149.

[140] Owens, J.A., A. Spirito, and M. McGuinn, *The Children's Sleep Habits Questionnaire (CSHQ): psychometric properties of a survey instrument for school-aged children.* Sleep New York, 2000. 23(8): pp. 1043–1052.

[141] Roid, G.H. and L.J. Miller, *Leiter International Performance Scale-Revised (Leiter-R).* 2011: Madrid: Psymtec.

[142] Harter, S., Self-Perception Profile for Children. 1983: University of Denver Press. Denver, ABD.

[143] Donders, J., D. DenBraber, and L. Vos, *Construct and criterion validity of the Behaviour Rating Inventory of Executive Function (BRIEF) in children referred for neuropsychological assessment after paediatric traumatic brain injury.* Journal of Neuropsychology, 2010. 4(2): pp. 197–209.

[144] Zimmerman, I.L., V.G. Steiner, and R.E. Pond, PLS-3: Preschool Language Scale-3. 1992: 2 Psychological Corporation. San Antonio, USA.

[145] Hidecker, M.J.C., et al., *Developing and validating the Communication Function Classification System for individuals with cerebral palsy.* Developmental Medicine & Child Neurology, 2011. 53(8): pp. 704–710.

[146] Fowler, E.G., et al., *Selective Control Assessment of the Lower Extremity (SCALE): development, validation, and interrater reliability of a clinical tool for patients with cerebral palsy.* Developmental Medicine & Child Neurology, 2009. 51(8): pp. 607–614.

[147] Sellers, D., et al., *Development and reliability of a system to classify the eating and drinking ability of people with cerebral palsy.* Developmental Medicine & Child Neurology, 2014. 56(3): pp. 245–251.

[148] Breau, L.M., et al., *Psychometric properties of the non-communicating children's pain checklist-revised.* Pain, 2002. 99(1): pp. 349–357.

[149] Swiggum, M., et al., *Pain in children with cerebral palsy: implications for pediatric physical therapy.* Pediatric Physical Therapy, 2010. 22(1): pp. 86–92.

Section 3

Therapies

Chapter 3

Current Rehabilitation Methods for Cerebral Palsy

Nilay Çömük Balcı

Additional information is available at the end of the chapter

http://dx.doi.org/10.5772/64373

Abstract

In rehabilitation of children with cerebral palsy (CP), varying approaches and techniques are used, ranging from very conservative and conventional techniques, such as muscle strengthening, manual stretching, and massage, to more complex motor learning-based theories, such as neurodevelopmental treatment, conductive education, and several others. The motor disorders seen in CP are frequently accompanied by disturbances of sensation, cognition, communication, perception, and/or behavior disorders; thus, therapy approaches are arranged to meet the individual child's needs. The approaches can be divided into two groups as with equipment and without equipment. Examples for without equipment rehabilitation approaches are neurodevelopmental treatment, conductive education constraint-induced movement therapy, and task-oriented therapy, whereas robotic therapy, virtual reality, and horse-back riding therapy are the examples of rehabilitation approaches with equipment. CP is a prevalent, disabling condition. Application of evidence-based methods ensures maximum gains in children. The concept that intense, task-specific exercises capitalize on the potential plasticity of the CNS and thus improve motor recovery has led to the development of several successful interventions for children with CP. Also approaches that improve the patient's motivation and target the activities of daily living and participation are the most effective approaches for functional recovery of the children with CP.

Keywords: cerebral palsy, rehabilitation, physiotherapy, current, present

1. Introduction

Cerebral palsy (CP) applies to an insult of the developing brain that produces a disorder of movement and posture. Primary symptoms of cerebral palsy are problems with muscle tone, balance, selectivity, and strength. Rehabilitation of the children with CP aims to reach and maintain optimal physical, sensory, intellectual, psychological, and social function. It includes providing the tools an individual needs to gain and maintain independence and self-determination. Brain plasticity is important to the pathophysiology and treatment of CP throughout a patient's life. This feature has directed research into functional recovery, and rehabilitation therapies that aim to capitalize on neuroplasticity are being developed. Recent recommendations state that intensive rehabilitation improves motor function in children with CP by including motor learning theories. Repetitive, goal-directed movements that are associated with sensory feedback and an attractive environment are likely to promote reorganization of the neuronal pathways and motor development after brain injuries [1, 2]. Advances in neuroscience suggest that the central nervous system (CNS) has some plasticity and the potential to reorganize throughout the entire lifespan rather than merely during a short period of development. Activity-dependent plasticity takes place in the motor cortex. The concept that intense, task-specific exercises capitalize on the potential plasticity of the CNS and thus improve motor recovery has led to the development of several successful interventions. In general, techniques used in CP rehabilitation can be classified as (1) approaches without using any equipment and (2) approaches with using equipments. In the rehabilitation of CP, there have been several major therapeutic practices during past years, including the Bobath concept and sensory integration; these models of treatment have been adopted as good practice and accepted as conventional approaches to treatment. Additional, well-controlled, randomized trials are needed to establish efficacy and to define the most appropriate roles for new technologies in physical rehabilitation interventions for children with CP [3, 4].

2. Approaches without using any equipment

2.1. Bobath concept

The Bobath approach, also known as neurodevelopmental treatment (NDT), was developed by Dr. Karel Bobath and Berta Bobath in the 1940s. The concept was based on observations of how abnormal tone interfered with the child's ability to develop functional activity. The Bobaths developed a theoretical framework for practice based on the neurophysiological knowledge of the day [5]. The Bobath concept says that normal quality of tone is necessary for effective movement. In Bobath concept, therapists use specialized handling techniques that improve the quality of tone and facilitate the movement patterns in the execution of everyday tasks. Also, active participation of the child is emphasized throughout treatment with the specific aim and controlling the activity. The quality of tone has always been central to this concept [6]. The Bobaths emphasized the need for movement strategies learnt in treatment to be carried over into everyday life activities. When planning the most appropriate activity, therapists draw on an in-depth knowledge of normal motor development and the control of movement [7]. NDT aims to normalize the muscle tone, inhibit primitive and abnormal reflexes, and to facilitate normal movements [8]. The Bobath concept based on the systems approach to motor control, with neuroplasticity as the primary mechanism for neurological recovery [9, 10]. Bobath concept helps to improve postural alignment and inhibit abnormal reflexes with child's active participation and practice of functional skills. Using handlings, the

http://dx.doi.org/10.5772/64373

therapist aims to facilitate the desired muscle action. Through these handlings, it is possible to conduct movements, influence muscle tone, and improve postural alignment and postural self-organization [11–13]. Self-organization facilitates posture and movement integration, allowing the use of postural control strategies contributing for motor learning and motor control improvement. Normal movements are facilitated, and abnormal patterns are inhibited to allow appropriate active reactions [14]. The therapist induces an expected motor response by means of the stimulation of sensory pathways, which are the gateways to motor control and motor learning [15, 16]. This approach also provides observation, analyzing a child's performance and finding his/her potential. The purpose of this approach is to correct abnormal postural tone and to facilitate more normal movement patterns for performing daily activities [17]. Despite the widespread use of NDT, studies of its effectiveness have reported conflicting or inconsistent findings. Thus, more accurate assessment tools are important for measuring the effectiveness of NDT in cerebral palsy (CP) rehabilitation [16].

2.2. Goal attainment therapy

The aim of this therapy for children with CP, as for most children with developmental disabilities, is to facilitate the child's participation in everyday life situations, e.g., to communicate with parents, siblings, and peers; to move from one place to another; to dress and undress; to eat; and to play. The choice of goals for therapy is dependent on many factors: the child's likings and the family's preferences, the society and environment in which the family lives, and the child's degree of disability [18, 19]. Gradually, a shift has occurred in therapy. Today the child is given the possibility to be more of an active problem solver (instead of, as previously, a passive recipient of treatment) in the context of the day-to-day environment. This treatment approach is referred to as 'task-oriented' approach and is built on theories of motor control. The development and learning of new skills occur in an interaction between the child, the task to be performed, and the particular environment in which the activity takes place [20–22]. This is the context in which the goals for therapy are set in close collaboration with the child's family and sometimes also the child. The goals and especially the grading of the goals in steps provide an individual plan for the child to learn the specific activity and reach the goal [23, 24]. Thus, it is important to integrate principles of motor learning in the treatment concept and adapt the principles to the prerequisites of each specific child. As CP is a very heterogeneous disorder, large differences exist between the children. Also from this viewpoint, the formulation of treatment goals offers an opportunity to an individualized treatment approach. The set goals should be specific, measurable, attainable, relevant, and timed (SMART) [25–31]. Functional training and practice of functional tasks are important parts of the rehabilitation management in CP. Achievement of functional goals was always the ultimate purpose of therapists [10]. Physiotherapists often identify a general aim in treatment of their patients, such as improving trunk balance or gait pattern. Such aims have general changes in the child's performance, they do not refer to a specific activity achievement. Setting a treatment goal involves identifying and formulating standards of motor activity, which are in advance of the child's current capacity. Previous studies on a group of quadriplegic children reported improved motor function after treatment using goal setting [32–35]. In randomized trials, the goal-directed therapy in real environment has been shown to be more effective than approaches focusing on impairments in quality of movement and muscle performance [35–38]. Collaborative goal setting and achieving meaningful, client-selected goals bring about effective therapy service [39, 40]. Effective listening and communication are strategies and fundamental components of successful interventions to establish a common goal [41, 42]. Treatment success was defined by Goal Attainment Scaling (GAS). GAS is an individualized criterion-referenced measurement that quantifies the achievement of treatment or intervention goals for different kinds of treatment issues [43, 44]. For each goal, client and therapist improved specific, observable, and quantifiable outcomes. Five outcome levels were identified, including expected level of performance (assigned 0), two levels of less favorable (assigned −2 or −1), and two levels of more favorable outcomes (assigned +1 or +2) [24].

2.3. Strength training programs

Enhancing muscular fitness and higher levels of muscular strength causes significantly better cardiometabolic risk factor profiles, lower risk of all-cause mortality, fewer cardiovascular disease events, and lower risk of developing functional limitations. In CP, muscle weakness is a primary impairment, and there is strong evidence showing that children with CP are significantly weaker than children with typical development [45–52]. In the past, strength training was considered to be contraindicated in children with CP because it was thought to increase muscles stiffness and result in an increase in spasticity. However, studies have found no change in spasticity during or after training, which supports the current belief that strength training for persons with spasticity is not contraindicated [53–55]. Muscle strength training studies have shown that training may strengthen muscles without adverse effects in children and adolescents with CP. The majority of participants were spastic diplegic or hemiplegic distribution. These trials are evidence for benefit of strength training programs that improve strength [56]. Also, there is an evidence that targeted strength training improves spasticity. Therefore, in conjunction with cardiorespiratory fitness, target muscle strengthening in children, adolescents, and adults with CP is imperative [57]. As for children with typical development, resistance training has observable benefits in strength among children, adolescents, and adults with CP [58]. There is inadequate evidence to show changes in activity or participating in everyday life. However, there are strong indications that strength training programs play an important role in the habilitation of individuals with CP [7]. Isokinetics has been used in testing and performance enhancement for over 30 years. In 1967, some authors introduced the concept of isokinetic exercise training and rehabilitation. Isokinetics are frequently chosen because of their inherent patient safety and objectivity. Isokinetic represents a match between mechanically imposed velocity and the subject movement that contacts against a controlled angular velocity. Therefore, through accommodating resistance, the muscle contracts at its maximal capability at all points throughout the range of motion [59]. Endurance exercises are considered as exercises that are done in a time limit of a person's ability to maintain either a specific force or power involving muscular contractions. Several studies have found out that endurance exercises can greatly increase strength in the muscles by adding specific weight training to their programs. Strength development through endurance training is important for the prevention and rehabilitation of injuries and for improving sport performance. Strength is also important for maintenance of functional capacity; with aging or injury, there is catabolic breakdown of the muscle connective tissue, resistance training presents the only natural method to offset such wasting conditions. Resistance exercise is a very common type of endurance training, which can improve the muscle strength and give a good balance to our bodies [60–65]. Strength training also increase the power of weak antagonist muscles and of the spastic agonists. Improvements with various modalities ranged from 19.6% with isokinetic strengthening to over 100% with training machines and free weights [66–70]. The nature of the relationship between strength and function is of considerable relevance to clinical practice. Task-oriented weight-bearing strength training for children with CP was effective in increasing strength and functional performance. Gains in strength improve functional motor performance, if strengthening exercises includes more functional closed kinetic chain exercises. In these exercises, the subject is weight bearing through the feet, and the body mass is raised and lowered over the feet by concentric and eccentric action of lower limb muscles, such as sit-to-stand and walking [71].

2.4. Conductive education

Conductive education (CE) is a combined educational and task-oriented approach for children with CP. Specially trained 'conductors' give education to homogeneous groups of children with motor disorders [72]. This approach has its origins in learning theory. The movement problems experienced by children with CP are thought of primary learning process problems. Training takes place in an educational setting. The conductor who is trained in all aspects of motor and cognitive development structures the activities, especially the self-care activities. Group work is important as a motivating factor, and there is a strong emphasis on the importance of anticipation, with forward planning of activities and volitional control in acquisition of new skills [73]. CE approach aims to educate people with physical disabilities to acquire new experiences in activities of daily living (ADLs). In this approach, the child is educated on how to use his/her abilities for performing active movements and generalizing this learning to different life situations. In this technique, children present activities in the form of a group, using music and rhythmic speech during activities. Paying attention to all aspect of child development, that is, the physical, intellectual, cognitive, and social approach, is important [74]. The CE approach is more effective in improving social interaction and relationships than the other approaches. Educational programs for parents can also improve the quality of life of children with CP in activities, such as eating, bowel, and urine control [75]. In Hungary, where this approach was pioneered, children tend to be in the educational setting all day. Frequently, group work and the use of specialized furniture are incorporated into more eclectic treatment programs [7]. Major differences in outcome between CE and another intensive rehabilitation program was not demonstrated [76]. A study comparing individual PT or OT with CE showed that CE improved coordinative hand functions and activities of daily living [77]. The emphasis of intervention is on independence in attaining goals rather than on quality of movement. CE is sometimes included in the group of complementary therapies for CP. It has been reported to be used by 21% of children with CP [6, 10, 78, 79].

2.5. Sensory Integration Training

Sensory integration therapy is based on the idea that some kids experience "sensory overload" and are oversensitive to certain types of stimulation. When children have sensory overload, their brains have trouble processing or filtering many sensations at once. Meanwhile, other children are undersensitive to some kinds of stimulation. Children who are undersensitive do not process sensory messages quickly or efficiently. These children may seem disconnected from their environment. In either case, children with sensory integration issues struggle to organize, understand, and respond to the information they take in from their surroundings. Sensory integration therapy exposes children to sensory stimulation in a structured, repetitive manner. The theory behind this treatment approach is that, over time, the brain will adapt and allow them to process and react to sensations more efficiently. CP has been treated with an emphasis on ameliorating motor impairments; however, more recently, the significant impact of concomitant sensory impairments has been acknowledged and targeted for evaluation and intervention. Sensory integration is developed by an occupational therapist, Jean Ayres, in the 1960s. In this concept, difficulties in planning and organizing behavior are attributed to problems of processing sensory inputs within the CNS, including vestibular, proprioceptive, tactile, visual, and auditory. Children with sensory integration dysfunction frequently use different sensory combination strategies. Treatment focuses on integration of neurological processing by facilitating the individual to process the type, quality, and intensity of sensation. Children with sensory integration problems often display inappropriate responses to sensory input. Some children show poor ability to register sensory information and therefore seek sensory input, and those who are hypersensitive to sensory stimuli require desensitizing. The processing of sensory information is fundamental for organizing behaviors. A significant number of children with CP have sensory impairments. Sensory integration may help processing and integration of this sensory information, thereby enhancing the child's acquisition of function [7, 80]. Programs of Sensory Integration Training in individuals and group treatments affect children with cerebral palsy. It was concluded that sensory integration training in children with cerebral palsy will be applied to combined programs and the relationship with individual and group treatments developed [81].

2.6. Constraint-induced movement therapy (CIMT)

Congenital hemiplegia is the most common form of unilateral CP, with a prevalence of 1 in 1300 live births. One side of the body has impairments in movement and/or sensation, which may cause difficulty with daily activities. The result of sensory and motor impairments often leads to "developmental disuse"—a phenomenon in which such children tend not to use the affected extremity, so it accordingly fails to develop [26, 82]. Constraint-induced movement therapy (CIMT) is specifically used to improve upper limb function in children with hemiplegia who account for approximately 30% of all children with CP [83]. CIMT aims to increase spontaneous use of the impaired arm by forcing the child to use it by restraining the other one. It is characterized by the following elements: restraining of the unaffected side, concentrated and intensive practice (over 2–3 treatment weeks for 6–7 days with the unaffected hand restrained 90% of the waking hours, followed by 10 days of a 6-hour intensive program), and shaping activities [84]. This protocol has been modified in a number of studies and more recent use with children with hemiplegia has featured a shorter duration of restraint (with none taking place at home) and the use of child-friendly treatment tasks [85]. One potential advantage of CIMT is that the restraint allows the therapist administering the intervention to focus solely on the more-affected arm [86]. Some clinical trials show that this modified CIMT significantly improves movement efficiency and bimanual arm use in hemiplegic children [87, 88]. A recent systematic review provides evidence of efficacy of CIMT for improving hand function. CIMT was initially used in adults with hemiparesis [89]. During the acute phase of stroke, the individual unable to use the upper limb effectively, which over time results in learned nonuse of the affected upper limb. Similar loss of function was found in children with hemiplegia [90–92]. During development, the children with hemiplegia frequently find that daily tasks are more effective and efficient using the nonaffected hand. CIMT increases functional ability in the affected upper limb with a concomitant cortical reorganization. In recent years, a variety of clinical trials bring out modified CIMT, where the unaffected limb is restrained for less than 3 hours a day. Restraint of the nonaffected limb may take several forms, including bivalved casts, a glove, or a sling. Activity programs involve selected tasks that are systematically increased in difficulty, this is often referred to as a shaping process. CIMT improves movement efficiency, performance, and perceived usage of the involved upper extremity hand and arm, the changes retains for 6 months. CIMT is efficacious in improving movement efficiency that was not age-dependent [88, 91–93]. CIMT is based on a concept that is not new but it is still experimental in hemiplegic CP. Further research is essential for its tolerability for children and families and to ensure that it is developmentally appropriate.

2.7. Bimanual training

The Bimanual training (BIT) provides bimanual training activities, which focus on improving the coordination of both arms using structured tasks in bimanual play and functional activities with intensive practice [94]. Historically, therapists have used a bimanual approach in the management of motor dysfunction in children with hemiplegia, but only recently has an intensive bimanual training program, the hand-arm bimanual intensive training (HABIT) been published to substantiate its effectiveness. This approach is based on motor learning theory (practice specificity, types of practice, and feedback), neuroplasticity (i.e., the potential of the brain to change by repetition, increasing movement complexity, motivation, and reward), and focuses on the equal use of both arms in bimanual tasks. Intensive BIT (e.g., HABIT), was developed with recognition that increased functional independence in the child's environment requires the combined use of both hands. BIT was developed in response to the limitations of CIMT, with a view to addressing bimanual coordination while maintaining the positive aspects of intensive training of the impaired arm. BIT also focuses on improving coordination of the two hands using structured task practice embedded in bimanual play and functional activities [86, 95, 96]. The lower extremity (LE) is generally less affected than the upper extremity (UE) in children with hemiplegic CP, normally allowing gait. However, impairments are observed in the involved LE ranging from isolated equines in the ankle to hip flexion and adduction with a fixed knee. In standing, children are unable to achieve postural symmetry, presenting an overload on one body side. This leads to limitations in walking abilities. In the past decade, intensive training techniques focusing on the UE (i.e., CIMT, intensive bimanual training) have shown tremendous promise in improving UE function. Hand-arm bimanual intensive therapy including lower extremities (HABIT-ILE) combines upper and lower bilateral extremity training [97, 98]. Frequently used bimanual tasks and activities are gross dexterity, manipulative games and tasks, functional tasks, arts and craft, and virtual reality (wii-fit, kinect). Frequently used bilateral lower extremity tasks are ball sitting, standing, balance board standing, virtual reality (wii-fit, kinect), walking/running, jumping, cycling, and making scooter. Bimanual activities that require trunk and LE postural adaptations are performed at a table of appropriate height (50% of the time) on unstable supports: sitting on fitness balls or standing on balance boards. Both the decreased time and the progressively increasing postural challenge represent the main difference from HABIT. Furthermore, 30% of the time is devoted to activities of daily living where standing and/or walking is required (dressing, brushing teeth, doing one's hair, transporting objects such as a tray, and household chores such as sweeping and washing dishes). Finally, the remaining time (20%) is spent in gross motor physical activities/play, such as bowling, ball playing, jumping rope, street hockey, use of wii-fit, balance bike (without pedals), scooter use, and wall climbing. These are performed in standing, walking, and running (or jumping) with the LE and simultaneously involving bimanual coordination. These activities are graded toward more demanding tasks for the LE [99].

2.8. Family-centered models

Family-centered care refers to how healthcare professionals interact and involve children's family in the care. A family-centered approach is characterized by therapist's practices that respect to families, where information is exchanged, where there is responsiveness to the family priorities and choices, and where family-therapist partnerships are fundamentally important. The family-centered practice has emphasis on child and family strengths rather than deficits. This approach facilitates family choice and control [100–103]. In this approach, effective intervention is based on collaborative decision making and respect for parents' understandings of their child's needs and appreciation of family and child worldviews, values, and preferences. Family-centered service promote the family's (including the child) self-determination, decision-making capabilities, and self-efficacy [104–107]. The principles underlying family-centered service include recognition of parents as the experts on their child's needs, the promotion of partnership, and support for the family's role in decision making for their child. There is evidence that family-centered care is related to physical or health benefits to children and psychosocial benefits for mothers [108]. Collaboration or a partnership between therapists and families has been endorsed as a best approach in the field of early intervention and pediatric rehabilitation [109–111]. Successful parent-therapist collaboration is characterized by the following therapist competencies: (1) ability to listen, share, and learn with families; (2) ability to foster the parental role and expertise; and (3) ability to facilitate parent-centered decision making about what is best for the child [42]. These abilities and behaviors, together, constitute the building blocks of family-centered service, effective help giving, and relationship-based practice [112, 113]. The "family-centred service" is built on three principles: (1) respect that parents know and want the best for their child, (2) every family is unique, and (3) optimal development occurs within a supportive family and a community context [18, 114, 115]. A family-centered service approach offers a perspective in which the child and biological aspects of the child are important but where the needs of the parents and the family are central to incorporate and support. The well-being of the family is essential to the well-being of the child. In many countries, (re)habilitation centers offer multiprofessional services to children with developmental disabilities, and a family-centered service approach is often an important basis in the work with families. Good team collaboration is needed to optimally coordinate services. Key features in this process are good organization and communication and a lucid process in the collaborative decision making when setting goals for therapy [116, 117].

3. Approaches with using equipments

3.1. Treadmill training

Approximately 41% of children with CP display limited walking ability. A typical form of gait training has been performed overground with assistive devices or parallel bars. The treadmill has recently gained more attention as an instrument for gait training and assessment with several advantages over conventional methods. The treadmill can help clinicians overcome space constraints, reduce physical demands, and establish a convenient set-up for gait evaluation [118]. Treadmill training is used for children with CP to help them to improve balance and build strength of their lower limbs so they could walk earlier and more efficiently than those children who did not receive treadmill training [65]. In recent years, there has been increasing interest in partial body weight-supported treadmill training (PBWSTT). In PBWSTT, the child is in a harness that supports their body weight, reducing some of the effort required for walking over the treadmill. The treadmill assists in production of steps while the child is supported in a safe environment. Recent studies have reported the benefits of gait training on a treadmill. Some studies showed that treadmill training helped children with cerebral palsy to walk about 101 days earlier than children who did not train by treadmill. A recent study, which looked at the effects of PBWSTT on endurance, functional gait, and balance, trained children for 30 minutes twice daily for 2 weeks, showed improvements in walking speed and energy efficiency. A recent systematic review of PBWSTT in young children with developmental disability (the majority of whom had CP) concluded that there was no definitive evidence that PBWSTT alone increases ambulatory ability. Although the systematic review did not support the effectiveness of the treatment, the evidence from some of the papers reviewed suggested some positive improvements [119, 120]. Positive effects of treadmill training were found in comparison with overground gait training on static and functional balance. The effects were found after 12 sessions of training at the aerobic threshold without body weight support. The benefits included an improvement in functional performance and greater independence in children with CP [121]. It is suggested that treadmill training may favor proprioceptive feedback, leading to adjustments for adequate postural balance and functional performance [122]. Also, backward walking (BW) training on the treadmill can improve the gross motor function measure, weight-bearing symmetry, and temporospatial gait parameters in individuals with spastic cerebral palsy. The muscles of the legs are active for a longer period during BW training when compared with forward (FW) training, and a longer period of muscle activity can result in greater muscle strength gain than with FW training. Furthermore, training in BW could require higher physiological and perceptual responses than FW at matched speed, as BW is the performance of a novel task for most children with CP. BW treadmill training helps children with spastic CP to improve walking capacity and decrease standing asymmetry of body weight distribution [123]. Treadmill gait training helps such children to repeat task-centered activities while walking; accordingly, they control velocity and develop a proper walking pattern by processing repeated sensory inputs obtained during walking. It is effective for increasing the muscular strength of the knee extensors and flexors as well as enhancing balance activities. Thus, it plays an important role in improving the functional activities of children with cerebral palsy. Enhanced muscular strength in the lower limbs causes adjusting the participants' posture, improving dynamic postural stability, and ultimately improving walking. Also, improved walking endurance and muscle strength leads to improved gait performance after treadmill training [124].

3.2. Robot-assisted therapy

Robot-assisted therapy (RAT) is conducted using robotic devices that enable the patients to perform specific limb movements. The main interest in using robots is to allow the patients to achieve a large amount of movement in a limited time. Additionally, the attractive human-machine interface has the capacity to motivate the child to perform his or her therapy through playful games, such as car races, or to perform exercises that mimic ADLs. Moreover, robotic devices allow the patient to receive visual, auditory, or sensory feedbacks. Finally, the robot gives performance-based assistance to the patients. This assistance can enhance the neuronal plasticity by enabling the patients to initiate and accomplish movements as actively as possible [125–132]. The strength of RAT is based on repetitive, goal-oriented, cognitive engaging tasks, which appear to be particularly interesting in the pediatric age, when the neuroplasticity is recognized to be at its maximum. Robotic therapy might increase functional strength and improve isolated movements. Because consistency of assistance can be maintained, intensity and difficulty can be set according to the patient's improvement. Several groups reported long-lasting improvements in standing and walking of children with CP. Also, parents and patients report improvements in terms of quality of life [133–135]. A device specifically developed for the locomotion training is the Lokomat (Hocoma, CH), made of two active orthoses, a weight-bearing system and a treadmill. This robotic rehabilitation has been proposed to improve walking and physical fitness [136]. It is reported that the muscular strength of ankle dorsi-flexion and plantarflexion increases in children with cerebral palsy who played a block break game and an airplane game using robotics in virtual reality three times per week for 12 weeks [137]. Robotic devices offer children fun and intensive rehabilitation that a human therapist cannot provide. These robots can be easily integrated as a relevant complement to therapy in the clinical setting. Studies have shown that combined passive and active training using a portable robot for children with CP is effective and feasible in a research laboratory and in a clinical setting. A repetitive, goal-directed, biofeedback training through motivating games in the laboratory and in the home environment is feasible. Robot-guided therapy can be an option for a home-based treatment program. The benefits of home-based robot-guided therapy are also similar to those of laboratory-based robot-guided therapy [138].

3.3. Virtual reality

Virtual reality has been defined as the use of interactive simulations created with computer to perform users in virtual environments that appear, sound, and feel similar to real-world objects and events [139, 140]. Users interact with virtual objects by moving and manipulating them. The therapeutic aims of virtual reality and interactive computer play are to provide users with more than just an entertaining experience [141]. The use of virtual reality in pediatric rehabilitation is based on its distinctive attributes that provide ecologically valid opportunities for active learning, which are enjoyable and motivating yet challenging and safe [142, 143]. Due to limitations in mobility and manual ability, children with CP may have fewer opportunities for free play. Without opportunities for self-initiated and spontaneous play, children can develop a learned helplessness and assume that they are unable to perform a task even though they may have the required physical abilities. In contrast to planned structured activities led by an adult, free play is characterized by children's spontaneous engagement in an activity that is intrinsically motivating and self-regulated [144]. Virtual reality can improve the patient's motivation and achievement in ADLs. Preliminary data suggest that this type of therapy also improves motor function in the upper and lower extremities that are caused by CP [127, 145]. The dynamic nature of stimulus increases the ability of cognitive and/or motor demands. The automated recording of task outcome enables clinicians to focus on child's performance within a virtual environment and to observe whether he or she is using effective strategies [146]. Clinicians can now design virtual environments to achieve a variety of therapeutic objectives by varying task complexity, type, and amount of feedback [147, 148]. The significance of virtual reality technology is related to the motivation it provides to perform multiple task-oriented repetitions [149]. Virtual reality is more important in children who are often not compliant in following a conventional exercise program because they find the exercises to be less interesting [150–153]. The technologies differ in both type and technical complexity. There are a variety of technologies that can be used to implement virtual environments. These include the use of standard desktop or laptop computer equipment, camera-based video capture gesture control devices (e.g., Microsoft's Kinect), Nintendo Wii Fit (http://wiifit.com/) head-mounted displays, haptic and other sensor- and/or actuator-based devices, and large screen immersive systems (e.g., Motek's CAREN http://www.motekmedical.com/) [153]. It is showed that children with a neurological gait disorder reported higher levels of motivation while gait training during a virtual reality soccer activity compared with training with therapy instruction [154, 155]. Participants' motivation levels were found to differ based on the type of virtual reality game played. Their motivation levels were less during a virtual reality navigation game than during conventional therapy and greater during virtual reality soccer than during conventional therapy. Finally, participants reported more fun and interest when doing dorsiflexion exercises in the context of GestureTek virtual reality games compared with completing exercises while sitting in a chair with therapist instruction. More specifically, 8 of 10 children increased their median energy expenditure significantly. Parents reported motivation-enabled performance, four participants self-reported feeling motivated, and volition levels were increased. Demonstration of the effectiveness of any virtual reality intervention depends on the degree to which the attained skills transfer to the "real world." Interactive computer play is one of the hottest areas in neurorehabilitation research, with much of the focus being on individuals with cerebral palsy [4, 156–158].

3.4. Cardiorespiratory endurance training

Many children, adolescents, and adults with CP have reduced cardiorespiratory endurance (the capacity of the body to perform physical activity that depends mainly on the aerobic or oxygen-requiring energy systems), muscle strength, and habitual physical activity participation [58]. Both reduced cardiorespiratory endurance and muscular weakness pose significant risks for negative health outcomes and early, cardiovascular, and all-cause mortality. Because people with CP have lower level muscle strength and cardiorespiratory endurance, they are at higher risk for developing cardiovascular diseases. This has been shown by increased cardiometabolic risk factors, including hypertension, cholesterol, HDL-C, visceral adipose tissue, and obesity in adults with CP [159–166]. Moreover, adults with CP, there were substantially increased estimates of chronic diseases, such as diabetes, asthma, hypertension and other cardiovascular conditions, stroke, joint pain, and arthritis [167]. In studies, the participants exercised at least two to four times per week for minimum 20 minutes and at a moderate intensity of about 60–75% maximum heart rate, 40–80% of heart rate reserve, or 50–65% peak oxygen uptake. The studies reported outcomes in aerobic performance, measured with an arm cranking/cycle test, and shuttle run test and in cardiorespiratory endurance [168–172].

Cardiorespiratory training can effectively increase cardiorespiratory endurance in children and young adults with CP. Exercise prescription for people with CP should include: (1) a minimum frequency of two to three times per week; (2) an intensity between 60 and 95% of peak heart rate, or between 40 and 80% of the HRR, or between 50 and 65% of VO2peak; and (3) a minimum time of 20 minutes per session, for at least 8 consecutive weeks, when training three times a week or for 16 consecutive weeks when training two times a week. Moreover, a pre-workout warm-up and cool-down could be added to reduce musculoskeletal injury [58]. A program of "functional exercises," combining aerobic and anaerobic capacity and strength training, in ambulatory children improves physical fitness and quality of life. Training programs on static bicycles or treadmill were beneficial for gait and gross motor development without enhancing spasticity and abnormal movement patterns [171, 173].

3.5. Hippotherapy

Hippotherapy is a rehabilitation strategy performed with a moving horse, which has demonstrated its potential to improve the mobility of children with CP. This therapy is designed to improve motor functioning and quality of movement in children with CP [174, 175]. The warmth and shape of the horse and the rhythmic, three-dimensional movement of horseback riding improve the flexibility, posture, balance, and mobility of the rider. Hippotherapy can be described as a low frequency, high repetition treatment strategy. Muscle contractions and postural adjustments are required to react to the horse's movements. A full-sized horse transfers about 110 multidimensional swinging motions to the rider each minute while walking. More specifically, in a 30-minute therapy session, a horse walking at a speed of 100 steps/minute will induce over 3000 steps. In order to maintain vertical alignment and react to these postural challenges, the child must engage their trunk muscles intensively. In most hippotherapy sessions, the child takes various positions (e.g., forward sitting, side sitting, and backward sitting). During the sessions, a therapist and a trained side walker provide support and movement possibilities for the child sitting on the horse. In addition, equine movement induces a scapular and pelvic dissociation in the rider, similar to what is observed in a normal gait pattern with asymmetric arm and pelvis movements [176, 177]. Horseback riding therapy reduces abnormal tone, promoting motor performance, creating symmetric alignment, and improving postural awareness, gait, and mobility. It is a walk practice for the upper body without the use of the legs. One systematic review and two meta-analyses provide evidence that hippotherapy positively affects postural control, balance, and muscle symmetry [178–180]. Session length ranged from 30 minutes to 1 hour with a frequency ranging from one to two sessions per week. According to a recent systematic review, a weekly 45-minute session of hippotherapy for 8–10 weeks was correlated with positive effects on gross motor function in children with CP [181]. The social functioning domain is influenced by various factors, such as education, socioeconomic status, cognition, communication abilities, and motor function [182]. The opportunity to use or practice communication, listening, and language skills during hippotherapy also results in the improvements in social functioning. Hippotherapy enhances the child's motivation and willingness for participation in an activity [183].

Author details

Nilay Çömük Balcı

Address all correspondence to: nlycmk@yahoo.com

Department of Physiotherapy and Rehabilitation, Faculty of Health Sciences, Baskent University, Ankara, Turkey

References

[1] Sakzewski L, Ziviani J, Boyd R. Systematic review and meta-analysis of therapeutic management of upper-limb dysfunction in children with congenital hemiplegia. Pediatrics. 2009;123:1111-1122. DOI:10.1542/peds.2008-3335.

[2] Holt RL, Mikati MA. Care for child development: basic science rationale and effects of interventions. Pediatric Neurology. 2011;44:239-253. DOI:10.1016/j.pediatrneurol.2010.11.009.

[3] Aisen ML, Kerkovich D, Mast J, Mulroy S, Wren TA, Kay RM, Rethlefsen SA. Cerebral palsy: clinical care and neurological rehabilitation. Lancet Neurology. 2011;10:844-852. DOI:10.1016/S1474-4422(11)70176-4.

[4] Tatla SK, Sauve K, Virji-Babul N, Holsti L, Butler C, Van Der Loos HF. Evidence for outcomes of motivational rehabilitation interventions for children and adolescents with cerebral palsy: an American Academy for Cerebral Palsy and Developmental Medicine systematic review. Developmental Medicine & Child Neurology. 2013;55:593-601. DOI: 10.1111/dmcn.12147.

[5] Mayston MJ. Physiotherapy management in cerebral palsy: an update on treatment approaches. In: Scrutton D, Damiano D, Mayston M, editors. Management of the motor disorders of children with cerebral palsy. 2nd ed. London: MacKieth Press, 2004. p. 147–160. No. 161. Clinics in developmental medicine.

[6] Mayston MJ. Setting the scene. In: Edwards S, editor. Neurological physiotherapy—a problem solving approach, 2nd ed. Edinburgh: Churchill Livingstone, 2002. p. 3–19.

[7] Barber CE. A guide to physiotherapy in cerebral palsy. Paediatrics and Child Health. 2008;18:410–413.

[8] Bobath B. The very early treatment of cerebral palsy. Developmental Medicine & Child Neurology. 1967;9:373–390.

[9] Fetters L, Kluzik J. The effects of neurodevelopmental treatment versus practice on the reaching of children with spastic cerebral palsy. Physical Therapy. 1996;76:346–358.

[10] Papavasiliou AS. Management of motor problems in cerebral palsy: a critical update for the clinician. European Journal of Paediatric Neurolology. 2009;13:387-396. DOI: 10.1016/j.ejpn.2008.07.009.

[11] Mayston M. Bobath concept: Bobath@ 50: Mid-life crisis—What of the future? Physiotherapy Research International. 2008;13:131–136.

[12] Velickovic TD, Perat MV. Basic principles of the neurodevelopmental treatment. Medicina, 2005;42:112–120.

[13] Howle J M. Neuro-developmental treatment approach: Theoretical foundations and principles of clinical practice. Osseum Entertainment; 2002.

[14] Ju YH, Hwang IS, Cherng RJ. Postural adjustment of children with spastic diplegic cerebral palsy during seated hand reaching in different directions. Archives of Physical Medicine and Rehabilitation. 2012; 93: 471.

[15] Tsorlakis N, Evaggelinou C, Grouios G, Tsorbatzoudis C. Effect of intensive neurodevelopmental treatment in gross motor function of children with cerebral palsy. Developmental Medicine & Child Neurology. 2004;46:740–745.

[16] Grazziotin Dos Santos C, Pagnussat AS, Simon AS, Py R, Pinho AS, Wagner MB. Humeral external rotation handling by using the Bobath concept approach affects trunk

extensor muscles electromyography in children with cerebral palsy. Research in Developmental Disabilities. 2014; 20:134-141. DOI: 10.1016/j.ridd.2014.09.013.

[17] Case-Smith J. Occupational therapy for children. 5th ed. St. Louis, MO: Mosby.

[18] Bamm EL, Rosenbaum P. Family-centred theory: origins, development, barriers, and supports to implementation in rehabilitation medicine. Archives of Physical Medicine and Rehabilitation. 2008;89:1618-1624.

[19] Nijhuis BJ, Reinders-Messelink HA, de Blecourt AC, Boonstra AM, Calame EH, Groothoff JW, Nakken H, Potema KL. Goal setting in Dutch paediatric rehabilitation. Are the needs and principal problems of children with cerebral palsy integrated into their rehabilitation goals? Clinical Rehabilitation. 2008;22:348-363.

[20] Valvano J. Activity-focused motor interventions for children with neurological conditions. Physical & Occupational Therapy in Pediatrics. 2004;24:79-107.

[21] Darrah J, Wiart L, Magill-Evans J. Do therapists' goals and interventions for children with cerebral palsy reflect principles in contemporary literature? Pediatric Physical Therapy. 2008; 20:334-339.

[22] Shumway-Cook A, Woollacott MH. Motor control: translating research into clinical practice. 3rd ed. Lippincott Williams and Wilkins; 2006.

[23] O'Neill DL, Harris SR. Developing goals and objectives for handicapped children. Physical Therapy. 1982;62:295-298.

[24] Hurn J, Kneebone I, Cropley M. Goal setting as an outcome measure: A systematic review. Clinical Rehabilitation. 2006;20:756-772.

[25] Van Duijenvoorde AC, Zanolie K, Rombouts SA, Raijmakers ME, Crone EA. Evaluating the negative or valuing the positive? Neural mechanisms supporting feedback-based learning across development. Journal of Neuroscience. 2008; 28:9495-9503.

[26] Stanley F, Blair E, Alberman E. Cerebral palsies: Epidemiology and causal pathways. London: Mac Keith Press; 2000.

[27] Palisano R, Rosenbaum P, Walter S, Russel D, Wood E, Galuppi B. Development and reliability of a system to classify gross motor function in children with cerebral palsy. Developmental Medicine & Child Neurology. 1997;39:214-223.

[28] Eliasson A, Rösblad B, Krumlinde-Sundholm L, Beckung E, Arner M, Ohrvall A, Rosenbaum P. Manual Ability Classification System (MACS) for children with cerebral palsy: scale development and evidence of validity and reliability. Developmental Medicine & Child Neurology. 2006;48:549-554.

[29] Law M, Darrah J, Pollock N, King G, Rosenbaum P, Russel D, Palisano R, Harris S, Armstrong R, Watt J. Family-centered functional therapy for children with cerebral palsy: An Emerging Practice Model. Physical & Occupational Therapy in Pediatrics. 1998;18:83-102.

[30] Siegert RJ, McPerson KM, Taylor WJ. Toward a cognitive-affective model of goal-setting in rehabilitation: is self-regulation theory a key step? Disability and Rehabilitation. 2004;26:1175-1183.

[31] Carlberg EB, Löwing K. Goal directed training in children with cerebral palsy. Turkish Journal of Medical Science, Pediatric Rehabilitation Special Issue. 2010;3:53-57.

[32] Bower E, Mc Lellan DL, Arney J, Campbell MJ. A randomised controlled trial of different intensities of physiotherapy and different goal-setting procedures in 44 children with cerebral palsy. Developmental Medicine & Child Neurology. 1996;38:226-237.

[33] Bower E. Goal setting and the measurement of change. In: Scrutton D, Damiano D, Mayston M, editors. Measurement of motor disorders in children with cerebral palsy. London: Mc Keith Press; 2004. p. 32-52.

[34] Bower E, Mc Lellan DL. Assessing motor skill acquisition in four centres for the treatment of children with cerebral palsy. Developmental Medicine & Child Neurology. 1994;36:902-909.

[35] Van den Broeck C, De Cat J, Molenaers G, Franki I, Himpens E, Severijns D, Desloovere K. The effect of individually defined physiotherapy in children with cerebral palsy (CP). European Journal of Paediatric Neurology. 2010;14:519-525. DOI:10.1016/j.ejpn. 2010.03.004.

[36] Novak I, Cusick A, Lannin N. Occupational therapy home programs for cerebral palsy: double-blind, randomized, controlled trial. Pediatrics. 2009;124:e606–e614.

[37] Ketelaar M, Vermeer A, Hart H, van Petegem-van Beek E, Helders PJ. Effects of a functional therapy program on motor abilities of children with cerebral palsy. Physical Therapy. 2001;81:1534–1545.

[38] Salem Y, Godwin EM. Effects of task-oriented training on mobility function in children with cerebral palsy. NeuroRehabilitation. 2009;24:307–313.

[39] Levack WM, Taylor K, Siegert RJ, Dean SG, McPherson KM, Weatherall M. Is goal planning in rehabilitation effective? A systematic review. Clinical Rehabilitation. 2006;20:739–755.

[40] Mastos M, Miller K, Eliasson AC, Imms C. Goal-directed training: linking theories of treatment to clinical practice for improved functional activities in daily life. Clinical Rehabilitation. 2007;21:47–55.

[41] King G, Currie M, Bartlett DJ, Gilpin M, Willoughby C, Tucker MA, Strachan D, Baxter D. The development of expertise in pediatric rehabilitation therapists: changes in approach, self-knowledge, and use of enabling and customizing strategies. Developmental Neurorehabilitation. 2007;10:223–240.

[42] Palisano RJ, Chiarello LA, King GA, Novak I, Stoner T, Fiss A. Participation-based therapy for children with physical disabilities. Disability and Rehabilitation. 2012;34:1041-1052. DOI:10.3109/09638288.2011.628740.

[43] Kirusek TJ, Smith A, Cardillo JE. Goals attainment scaling: applications, theory and measurement. Hillsdale, New Jersey: Laurence Erlbaum Associates; 1994.

[44] Palisano RJ. Validity of goal attainment scaling in infants with motor delays. Physical Therapy. 1993;73:651-660.

[45] Wiley ME, Damiano DL. Lower-extremity strength profiles in spastic cerebral palsy. Developmental Medicine & Child Neurology. 1998;40: 100–107.

[46] Eek MN, Tranberg R, Beckung E. Muscle strength and kinetic gait pattern in children with bilateral spastic CP. Gait & Posture. 2011; 33: 333–337.

[47] Williams MA, Haskell WL, Ades PA, Amsterdam EA, Bittner V, Franklin BA, Gulanick M, Laing ST, Stewart KJ. Resistance exercise in individuals with and without cardiovascular disease: 2007 update: a scientific statement from the American Heart Association Council on Clinical Cardiology and Council on Nutrition, Physical Activity, and Metabolism. Circulation. 2007;116:572–584.

[48] Jurca R, Lamonte MJ, Church TS, Earnest CP, Fitzgerald SJ, Barlow CE, Jordan AN, Kampert JB, Blair SN. Associations of muscle strength and fitness with metabolic syndrome in men. Medicine & Science in Sports & Exercise. 2004; 36: 1301–1307.

[49] Jurca R, Lamonte MJ, Barlow CE, Kampert JB, Church TS, Blair SN. Association of muscular strength with incidence of metabolic syndrome in men. Medicine & Science in Sports & Exercise. 2005; 37:1849–1855.

[50] Peterson MD, Saltarelli WA, Visich PS, Gordon PM. Strength capacity and cardiometabolic risk clustering in adolescents. Pediatrics. 2014;133: e896–e903.

[51] Gale CR, Martyn CN, Cooper C, Sayer AA. Grip strength, body composition, and mortality. International Journal of Epidemiology 2007;36:228–235.

[52] Brill PA, Macera CA, Davis DR, Blair SN, Gordon N. Muscular strength and physical function. Medicine & Science in Sports & Exercise. 2000;32:412–416.

[53] Damiano DL, Vaughan CL, Abel MF. Muscle response to heavy resistance exercise in children with spastic cerebral palsy. Developmental Medicine & Child Neurology. 1995;37:731–739.

[54] Scholtes VA, Becher JG, Comuth A, Dekkers H, Van Dijk L, Dallmeijer AJ. Effectiveness of functional progressive resistance exercise strength training on muscle strength and mobility in children with cerebral palsy: a randomized controlled trial. Developmental Medicine & Child Neurology. 2010;52:e107–e113.

[55] Morton JF, Brownlee M, McFadyen AK. The effects of progressive resistance training for children with cerebral palsy. Clinical Rehabilitation. 2005;19 283–289.

[56] Dodd KJ, Taylor NF, Damiano DL. A systematic review of the effectiveness of strength training programs for people with cerebral palsy. Archives of Physical Medicine and Rehabilitation.2002; 83:1157–1164.

[57] Engsberg JR, Ross SA, Collins DR. Increasing ankle strength to improve gait and function in children with cerebral palsy: a pilot study. Pediatric Physical Therapy. 2006;18:266–275.

[58] Verschuren O, Peterson MD, Balemans AC, Hurvitz EA. Exercise and physical activity recommendations for people with cerebral palsy. Developmental Medicine & Child Neurology. 2016; 7. DOI: 10.1111/dmcn.13053.

[59] Davis B, Bull R, Roscoe Roscoe D. Physical education and the study of sport. 4th ed. Edinburgh: Mosby; 2000. p. 130–1150.

[60] Brandom R. Physical medicine and rehabilitation. 2nd ed. Philadelphia: Harcourt Health Science Company; 2000. p. 400–404.

[61] Mccall G, Byrnes W, Dickinson A, Pattany P, Fleck SJ. Muscle fiber hypertrophy, hyperplasia, and capillary density in college men after resistance training. Journal of Applied Physiology. 1996;81:2004–2010.

[62] Graham A, Reid A. Physical fitness of adults with an intellectual disability: A 13-year follow-up study. Research Quarterly for Exercise and Sport. 2000;71:152–161.

[63] Sutherland DH, Davis JR. Common abnormalities of the knee in cerebral palsy. Clinical Orthopaedics and Related Research. 1993;288:139–147.

[64] Carmeli E, Barchad S, Masharawi Y, Coleman R. Impact of a walking program in people with Down syndrome. Journal of Strength and Conditioning Research. 2004;18:180–184.

[65] Olama KA. Endurance exercises versus treadmill training in improving muscle strength and functional activities in hemiparetic cerebral palsy. Egyptian Journal of Medical Human Genetics. 2011;12:193-199.

[66] Damiano DL, Kelly LE, Vaughan CL. Effects of a quadriceps femoris strengthening programme on crouch gait in children with cerebral palsy. Physical Therapy. 1995;75:658–667.

[67] MacPhail HEA, Kramer JF. Effect of isokinetic strength training on functional ability and walking efficiency in adolescents with cerebral palsy. Developmental Medicine & Child Neurology. 1995;37:763–775.

[68] Damiano DL, Abel MF. Functional outcomes of strength training in spastic cerebral palsy. Archives of Physical Medicine and Rehabilitation.1998;79:119–125.

[69] Dodd KJ, Taylor NF, Graham HK. A randomized clinical trial of strength training in young people with cerebral palsy. Developmental Medicine & Child Neurology. 2003;45:652–657.

[70] Horvat M. Effects of a progressive resistance training program on an individual with spastic cerebral palsy. American Corrective Therapy Journal. 1987;41:7–11.

[71] Blundell SW, Shepherd RB, Dean CM, Adams RD. Functional strength training in cerebral palsy: a pilot study of a group circuit training class for children aged 4–8 years. Clinical Rehabilitation. 2003;17:48–57.

[72] Bairstow P, Cochrane R. Is conductive education transplantable? British Journal of Special Education. 1993;20:84–88.

[73] Medveczky E. Conductive education as an educational method of neurorehabilitation. Budapest: International Petö Institute; 2006.

[74] Hari M. The human principle in conductive education. Peto Magazine; 1996. p. 9–12.

[75] Dalvand H, Dehghan L, Feizy A, Amirsalai S, Bagheri H. Effect of the Bobath technique, conductive education and education to parents in activities of daily living in children with cerebral palsy in Iran. Hong Kong Journal of Occupational Therapy. 2009; 19:14-19.

[76] Odman PE, Oberg BE. Effectiveness and expectations of intensive training: a comparison between child and youth rehabilitation and conductive education. Disability and Rehabilitation. 2006; 28:561–570.

[77] Blank R, von Kries R, Hesse S, von Voss H. Conductive education for children with cerebral palsy: effects on hand motor functions relevant to activities of daily living. Archives of Physical Medicine and Rehabilitation. 2008;89:251–259.

[78] Parkes J, Donnelly M, Dolk H, Hill N. Use of physiotherapy and alternatives by children with cerebral palsy: a population study. Child Care Health & Development. 2002;28:469–477.

[79] Liptak GS. Complementary and alternative therapies for cerebral palsy. Mental Retardation and Developmental Disabilities Research Reviews. 2005;11:156–163.

[80] Spitzer S, Roley SS. Sensory integration revisited. In: Roley SS, Blanche EI, Schaaf RC, editors. Understanding the nature of sensory integration with diverse populations. Therapy Skills Builders; 2001. p. 3–27.

[81] Bumin G, Kayihan H. Effectiveness of two different sensory-integration programmes for children with spastic diplegic cerebral palsy. Disability and Rehabilitation. 2001;23:394-399.

[82] Charles J, Gordon AM. A critical review of constraint-induced movement therapy and forced use in children with hemiplegia. Neural Plasticity. 2005;12:245–261.

[83] Hagberg B, Hagberg G, Beckung E, Uverbrant P. Changing panorama of cerebral palsy in Sweden VIII. Prevalence and origin in the birth year period 1991–1994. Acta Paediatrica. 2001; 90: 271–277.

[84] Taub E, Wolf SL. Constraint induction techniques to facilitate upper extremity use in stroke patients. Topics in Stroke Rehabilitation. 1997;3:1–24.

[85] Gordon AM, Charles JR, Wolf SL. Methods of constraint induced movement therapy for children with hemiplegic cerebral palsy: Development of a child-friendly intervention for improving upper-extremity function. Archives of Physical Medicine and Rehabilitation. 2005;86:837–844.

[86] Dong VA, Tung IH, Siu HW, Fong KN. Studies comparing the efficacy of constraint-induced movement therapy and bimanual training in children with unilateral cerebral palsy: a systematic review. Developmental Neurorehabilitation. 2013;16:133-143. DOI: 10.3109/17518423.2012.702136.

[87] Eliasson AC, Sundholm LK, Shaw K, Wang C. Effects of constraint-induced movement therapy in young children with hemiplegic cerebral palsy: An adapted model. Developmental Medicine & Child Neurology. 2005;47:266–275.

[88] Charles JR, Wolf SL, Schneider JA, Gordon AM. Efficacy of a child-friendly form of constraint-induced movement therapy in hemiplegic cerebral palsy: A randomized control trial. Developmental Medicine & Child Neurology. 2006;48:635–642.

[89] Novak I, McIntyre S, Morgan C, Campbell L, Dark L, Morton N, Stumbles E, Wilson SA, Goldsmith S. A systematic review of interventions for children with cerebral palsy: State of the evidence. Developmental Medicine & Child Neurology. 2013; 55:885–910.

[90] Taub E. Somatosensory deafferentation research with monkeys: implications for rehabilitation medicine. In: Ince LP, editor. Behavioural psychorehabilitation medicine; clinical applications. Philadelphia: Williams and Wilkins; 1980. p. 371–401.

[91] Deluca SC, Echols K, Law CR, Ramey SL. Intensive paediatric constraint-induced therapy for children with cerebral palsy: randomized, controlled, crossover trial. Journal of Child Neurology. 2006;21:931–938.

[92] Hoare B, Imms C, Carey L, Wasiak J. Constraint induced movement therapy in the treatment of the upper limb in children with hemiplegic cerebral palsy: a cochrane systematic review. Clinical Rehabilitation. 2007;21:675–685.

[93] Gordon AM, Charles J, Wolf SL. Efficacy of constraint-induced movement therapy on involved upper-extremity use in children with hemiplegic cerebral palsy is not age-dependent. Pediatrics. 2006;117:363–373.

[94] Gordon AM, Schneider JA, Chinnan A, Charles JR. Efficacy of a hand-arm bimanual intensive therapy (HABIT) in children with hemiplegic cerebral palsy: A randomized control trial. Developmental Medicine & Child Neurology. 2007;49:830–838.

[95] Nudo RJ. Adaptive plasticity in motor cortex: Implications for rehabilitation after brain injury. Journal of Rehabilitation Medicine. 2003;41:7–10.

[96] Kleim JA, Hogg TM, VandenBerg PM, Cooper NR, Bruneau R, Remple M. Cortical synaptogenesis and motor map reorganization occur during late, but not early, phase of motor skill learning. Journal of Neuroscience 2004;24:628–633.

[97] Caty GD, Arnould C, Thonnard JL, Lejeune TM. ABILOCO-Kids: A Rasch-built 10-item questionnaire for assessing locomotion ability in children with cerebral palsy. Journal of Rehabilitation Medicine. 2008;40:823–830.

[98] Domagalska ME, Szopa AJ, Lembert DT. A descriptive analysis of abnormal postural patterns in children with hemiplegic cerebral palsy. Medical Science Monitor. 2011;17: CR110–CR116.

[99] Bleyenheuft Y, Gordon AM. Hand-arm bimanual intensive therapy including lower extremities (HABIT-ILE) for children with cerebral palsy. Physical and Occupational Therapy in Pediatrics. 2014;34:390-403. DOI: 10.3109/01942638.2014.932884.

[100] Dunst CJ, Trivette CM. Meta-analytic structural equation modeling of the influences of family-centered care on parent and child psychological health. International Journal of Pediatrics. 2009;2009:1-9.

[101] Dunst CJ, Trivette CM, Hamby DW. Meta-analysis of family-centered help-giving practices research. Mental Retardation and Developmental Disabilities Research Reviews. 2007;13:370-378.

[102] Chiarello L. Family-centered care. In: Effgen S, editor. Meeting the physical therapy needs of children. 2nd ed. Philadelphia, PA: F.A. Davis; 2013.p.153-180.

[103] King G, Chiarello L. Family-centered care for children with cerebral palsy: conceptual and practical considerations to advance care and practice. Journal of Child Neurology. 2014;29:1046-1054. DOI: 10.1177/0883073814533009.

[104] Wampold BE. The great psychotherapy debate: Models, methods, and findings. Mahwah, NJ: Lawrence Erlbaum; 2001.

[105] Franck LS, Callery P. Re-thinking family-centred care across the continuum of children's healthcare. Child Care Health and Development. 2004;30:265–277.

[106] Rosenbaum P, King S, Law M, King G, Evans J. Family-centred service: A conceptual framework and research review. Physical and Occupational Therapy in Pediatrics. 1998;18:1–20.

[107] Johns N, Harvey C. Training for work with parents: Strategies for engaging practitioners who are uninterested or resistant. Infants & Young Children. 1993;5:52–57.

[108] King S, Teplicky R, King G, Rosenbaum P. Family-centered service for children with cerebral palsy and their families: a review of the literature. Seminars in Pediatric Neurology. 2004;11:78–86.

[109] Moore TG, Larkin H. "More than my child's disability": A comprehensive review of family-centred practice and family experiences of early childhood intervention services. Melbourne: Scope (Vic) Inc.; 2006.

[110] Bailey DB Jr, Buysse V, Edmondson R, Smith TM. Creating family-centered services in early intervention: perceptions of professionals in four states. Exceptional Children. 1992;58:298–309.

[111] Kalmanson B, Seligman S. Family-provider relationships: The basis of all interventions. Infants & Young Children. 1992;4:46–52.

[112] Dunst CJ, Trivette CM. Empowerment, effective help-giving practices and family-centered care. Pediatric Nursing. 1996;22:334–337

[113] King G, King SM, Rosenbaum PL. Interpersonal aspects of care-giving and client outcomes: A review of the literature. Ambulatory Children Health. 1996;2:151–160.

[114] Rosenbaum P. Families and service providers: Forging effective connections, and why it matters. In: Scrutton D, Damiano D, Mayston M, editors. Management of the motor disorders of children with cerebral palsy. 2nd ed. Clinics In Developmental Medicine No. 161. London: Mac Keith Press; 2004. p.22-31.

[115] Wiart L, Ray L, Darrah J, Magill-Evans J. Parents' perspectives on occupational therapy and physical therapy goals for children with cerebral palsy. Disability and Rehabilitation. 2010;32:248–258.

[116] Preston KM. A team approach to rehabilitation. Home Healthcare Nurse. 1990;8:17-23.

[117] Nijhuis BJ, Reinders-Messelink HA, de Blécourt AC, Hitters WM, Groothoff JW, Nakken H, Postema K. Family-centred care in family-specific teams. Clinical Rehabilitation. 2007;21:660-671.

[118] Jung T, Kim Y, Kelly LE, Abel MF. Biomechanical and perceived differences between overground and treadmill walking in children with cerebral palsy. Gait & Posture. 2016;45:1-6. DOI: 10.1016/j.gaitpost.2015.12.004.

[119] Provost B, Dieruf K, Burtner PA, Phillips JP, Bernitsky-Beddingfield A, Sullivan KJ, Bowen CA, Toser L. Endurance and gait in children with cerebral palsy after intensive body weight-supported treadmill training. Pediatric Physical Therapy. 2007;19:2–10.

[120] Laforme Fiss AC, Effgen SK. Outcomes for young children with disabilities associated with the use of partial, body-weight supported, treadmill training: an evidence-based review. Physical Therapy Reviews. 2006;11:179–189.

[121] Grecco LA, Tomita SM, Christovão TC, Pasini H, Sampaio LM, Oliveira CS.. Effect of treadmill gait training on static and functional balance in children with cerebral palsy: a randomized controlled trial. Brazilian journal of physical therapy. 2013;17:17–23.

[122] Marchese R, Diverio M, Zucchi F, Lentino C, Abbruzzese G. The role of sensory cues in the rehabilitation of parkinsonian patients: a comparison of two physical therapy protocols. Movement Disorders. 2000;15:879–883.

[123] Kim SG, Ryu YU, Je HD, Jeong JH, Kim HD. Backward walking treadmill therapy can improve walking ability in children with spastic cerebral palsy: a pilot study. International Journal of Rehabilitation Research. 2013;36:246-252. DOI: 10.1097/MRR.0b013e32835dd620.

[124] Cho C, Hwang W, Hwang S, Chung Y. Treadmill training with virtual reality improves gait, balance, and muscle strength in children with cerebral palsy. The Tohoku Journal of Experimental Medicine. 2016;238:213-218. DOI: 10.1620/tjem.238.213.

[125] Fasoli SE, Fragala-Pinkham M, Hughes R, Hogan N, Krebs HI, Stein J. Upper limb robotic therapy for children with hemiplegia. American Journal of Physical Medicine and Rehabilitation. 2008;87:929-936.

[126] Fasoli SE, Ladenheim B, Mast J, Krebs HI. New horizons for robot-assisted therapy in pediatrics. American Journal of Physical Medicine and Rehabilitation. 2012;91:280-289.

[127] Fluet GG, Qiu Q, Kelly D, Parikh HD, Ramirez D, Saleh S, Adamovich SV. Interfacing a haptic robotic system with complex virtual environments to treat impaired upper extremity motor function in children with cerebral palsy. Developmental Neurorehabilitation. 2010;13:335-345. DOI: 10.3109/17518423.2010.501362.

[128] Frascarelli F, Masia L, Di Rosa G, Cappa P, Petrarca M, Castelli E, Krebs HI. The impact of robotic rehabilitation in children with acquired or congenital movement disorders. European Journal of Physical and Rehabilitation Medicine. 2009;45:135-141.

[129] Pignolo L. Robotics in neuro-rehabilitation. Journal of Rehabilitation Medicine. 2009;41:955-960.

[130] Krebs HI, Palazzolo JJ, Dipietro L. Rehabilitation robotics: performance-based progressive robot-assisted therapy. Autonomous Robots. 2003;15:7-20.

[131] Sapin J. Conception d'un robot interactif pour la re-education des membres supérieurs de patients cérébrolésés [thesis]. Louvain-la-Neuve, Belgium: Université catholique de Louvain; 2010.

[132] Gilliaux M, Renders A, Dispa D, Holvoet D, Sapin J, Dehez B, Detrembleur C,Lejeune TM, Stoquart G. Upper limb robot-assisted therapy in cerebral palsy: a single-blind randomized controlled trial. Neurorehabilitation and Neural Repair. 2015;29:183-192. DOI: 10.1177/1545968314541172.

[133] Meyer-Heim A, Ammann-Reiffer C, Schmartz A, Schafer J, Sennhauser FH, Heinen F, Knecht B, Dabrowski E, Borggraefe I. Improvement of walking abilities after robotic-assisted locomotion training in children with cerebral palsy. Archives of Disease in Childhood. 2009;94(8):615-620. DOI: 10.1136/adc.2008.145458.

[134] Borggraefe I, Kiwull L, Schaefer JS, Koerte I, Blaschek A, Meyer-Heim A, Heinen F. Sustainability of motor performance after robotic-assisted treadmill therapy in children: An open, non-randomized baseline-treatment study. European Journal of Physical Rehabilitation and Medicine. 2010;46:125-131.

[135] Borggraefe I, Schaefer JS, Klaiber M, Dabrowski E, Ammann-Reiffer C, Knecht B, Berweck S, Heinen F, Meyer-Heim A. Robotic-assisted treadmill therapy improves walking and standing performance in children and adolescents with cerebral palsy. European Journal of Paediatric Neurology. 2010;14:496-502.

[136] Peri E, Biffi E, Maghini C, Marzorati M, Diella E, Pedrocchi A, Turconi AC,Reni G. An ecological evaluation of the metabolic benefits due to robot-assisted gait training. Annual International Conference of the IEEE Engineering in Medicine and Biology Society. 2015;2015:3590-3593. DOI:10.1109/EMBC.2015.7319169.

[137] Burdea GC, Cioi D, Kale A, Janes WE, Ross SA, Engsberg JR. Robotics and gaming to improve ankle strength, motor control, and function in children with cerebral palsy: a case study series. IEEE Transactions on Neural Systems and Rehabilitation Engineering. 2013;21:165-173.

[138] Chen K, Wu YN, Ren Y, Liu L, Gaebler-Spira D, Tankard K, Lee J, Song W, Wang M, Zhang LQ. Home-based versus laboratory-based robotic ankle training for children with cerebral palsy: A pilot randomized comparative trial. Archives of Physical Medicine and Rehabilitation. 2016 Feb 19. PII: S0003-9993(16)00104-0. DOI: 10.1016/j.apmr.2016.01.029.

[139] Rizzo AA. Virtual reality and disability: emergence and challenge. Disability and Rehabilitation. 2002;24:567-569.

[140] Sandlund M, McDonough S, Hager-Ross C. Interactive computer play in rehabilitation of children with sensorimotor disorders: a systematic review. Developmental Medicine & Child Neurology. 2009;51:173-179.

[141] Weiss PL, Tirosh E, Fehlings D. Role of virtual reality for cerebral palsy management. Journal of Child Neurology. 2014;29:1119-1124.DOI: 10.1177/0883073814533007.

[142] Schultheis MT, Rizzo AA. The application of virtual reality technology for rehabilitation. Rehabilitation Psychology. 2001;46:296-311.

[143] Lange B, Flynn SM, Rizzo AA. Game-based tele-rehabilitation. European Journal of Physical Rehabilitation Medicine. 2009;45:143-151.

[144] Rios-Rincon AM, Adams K, Magill-Evans J, Cook A. Playfulness in children with limited motor abilities when using a robot. Physical and Occupational Therapy in Pediatrics. 2015;13:1-15.

[145] Wu YN, Hwang M, Ren Y, Gaebler-Spira D, Zhang LQ. Combined passive stretching and active movement rehabilitation of lower-limb impairments in children with

cerebral palsy using a portable robot. Neurorehabilitation and Neural Repair. 2011; 25:378–385.

[146] Snider L, Majnemer A. Virtual reality as a therapeutic modality for children with cerebral palsy. Developmental Neurorehabilitation. 2010;13:120-128.

[147] Kizony R, Weiss PL, Rand D. Designing and adapting VR technology and VEs for rehabilitation: a multidisciplinary approach. In: Cobb S, Lange B, editors. Virtual reality technologies for health and clinical applications, Vol. 4: Design, technologies, tools, methodologies & analysis. New York: Springer. In press.

[148] Levin ML, Deutsch J, Kafri M, et al. Validity of virtual reality environments for motor rehabilitation. In: Weiss PL, Keshner EA, Levin MF, eds. Virtual reality technologies for health and clinical applications, Vol. 1: Applying virtual reality technologies to motor rehabilitation. New York: Springer. In press.

[149] Page SJ, Levine P, Sisto S, Bond Q, Johnston MV. Stroke patients' and therapists' opinions of constraint-induced movement therapy. Clinical Rehabilitation. 2002;16:55-60.

[150] Rizzo AA, Kim G. A SWOT analysis of the field of virtual rehabilitation and therapy. Presence. 2005;14:1-28.

[151] Laufer Y, Weiss PL. Virtual reality in the assessment and treatment of children with motor impairment: a systematic review. Journal of Physical Therapy Education. 2011;25:59-71.

[152] Saposnik G, Levin MF. Virtual reality in stroke rehabilitation: a meta-analysis and implications for clinicians. Stroke. 2011;42:1380-1386.

[153] Weiss PL, Weintraub N, Laufer Y. Virtual reality therapy in pediatric rehabilitation. In: Chau T, editor. Pediatric rehabilitation engineering: From disability to possibility, London: Taylor & Francis; 2011.p.291-328.

[154] Brutsch K, Koenig A, Zimmerli L, Mérillat-Koeneke S, Riener R, Jäncke L, van Hedel HJA, Meyer-Heim A. Virtual reality for enhancement of robot-assisted gait training in children with central gait disorders. Journal of Rehabilitation Medicine. 2011;43:493–499.

[155] Brütsch K, Schuler T, Koenig A, Zimmerli L, Koeneke SM, Lünenburger L, Riener R, Jäncke L, Meyer-Heim A. Influence of virtual reality soccer game on walking performance in robotic assisted gait training for children. Journal of Neuroengineering and Rehabilitation. 2010;7:15.

[156] Sandlund M, Waterworth EL, Hager C. Using motion interactive games to promote physical activity and enhance motor performance in children with cerebral palsy. Developmental Neurorehabilitation. 2011;14:15–21.

[157] Jannink MJ, van der Wilden GJ, Navis DW, Visser G, Gussinklo J, Ijzerman M. A low-cost video game applied for training of upper extremity function in children with cerebral palsy: a pilot study. Cyberpsychology & Behavior. 2008;11:27-32

[158] Harris K, Reid D. The influence of virtual reality play on children's motivation. Canadian Journal of Occupational Therapy. 2005;72:21–29.

[159] Myers J, Prakash M, Froelicher VF, Do D, Partington S, Atwood JE. Exercise capacity and mortality among men referred for exercise testing. The New England Journal of Medicine. 2002;346:793–801.

[160] Blair SN, Cheng Y, Holder JS. Is physical activity or physical fitness more important in defining health benefits? Medicine and Science in Sports and Exercise. 2001;33:379–399.

[161] Artero EG, Lee DC, Ruiz JR, Sui X, Ortega FB, Church TS, Lavie CJ, Castillo MJ, Blair SN. A prospective study of muscular strength and all-cause mortality in men with hypertension. Journal of the American College of Cardiology. 2011;57:1831–1837.

[162] Ortega FB, Silventoinen K, Tynelius P, Rasmussen F. Muscular strength in male adolescents and premature death: cohort study of one million participants. BMJ. 2012;345:e7279.

[163] Peterson M, Zhang P, Haapala H, Wang S, Hurvitz E. Greater adipose tissue distribution and diminished spinal musculoskeletal density in adults with cerebral palsy. Archives of Physical Medicine and Rehabilitation. 2015;96:1828–1833.

[164] Peterson MD, Haapala HJ, Hurvitz EA. Predictors of cardiometabolic risk among adults with cerebral palsy. Archives Physical Medicine and Rehabilitation. 2012;93:816–821.

[165] van der Slot WM, Roebroeck ME, Nieuwenhuijsen C, Bergen MP, Stam HJ, Burdorf A, van den Berg-Emons RJ, Move Fit and Lifespan Research Group. Cardiovascular disease risk in adults with spastic bilateral cerebral palsy. Journal of Rehabilitation Medicine. 2013;45:866–872.

[166] Ryan JM, Crowley VE, Hensey O, McGahey A, Gormley J. Waist circumference provides an indication of numerous cardiometabolic risk factors in adults with cerebral palsy. Archives of Physical Medicine and Rehabilitation. 2014;95:1540–1546.

[167] Peterson MD, Ryan JM, Hurvitz EA, Mahmoudi E. Chronic conditions in adults with cerebral palsy. JAMA. 2015;314:2303–2305.

[168] Nsenga AL, Shephard RJ, Ahmaidi S. Aerobic training in children with cerebral palsy. International Journal of Sports Medicine. 2013;34:533–537.

[169] Unnithan VB, Katsimanis G, Evangelinou C, Kosmas C, Kandrali I, Kellis E. Effect of strength and aerobic training in children with cerebral palsy. Medicine and Science in Sports and Exercise. 2007;39:1902–1909.

[170] van den Berg-Emons RJ, van Baak MA, Speth L, Saris WH. Physical training of school children with spastic cerebral palsy: effects on daily activity, fat mass and fitness. International Journal of Rehabilitation Research. 1998;21:179–194.

[171] Verschuren O, Ketelaar M, Gorter JW, Helders PJ, Uiterwaal CS, Takken T. Exercise training program in children and adolescents with cerebral palsy: a randomized controlled trial. Archives of Pediatrics & Adolescent Medicine. 2007;161:1075–1081.

[172] Slaman J, Roebroeck M, van der Slot W, Twisk J, Wensink A, Stam H, van den Berg-Emons R. LEARN 2 MOVE Research Group. Can a lifestyle intervention improve physical fitness in adolescents and young adults with spastic cerebral palsy? A randomized controlled trial. Archives of Physical Medicine and Rehabilitation. 2014;95:1646–1655.

[173] Williams H, Pountney T. Effects of a static bicycling programme on the functional ability of young people with cerebral palsy who are non-ambulant. Developmental Medicine and Child Neurology. 2007;49:522–527.

[174] Kavanagh J, Barrett R, Morrison S. Age-related differences in head and trunk coordination during walking. Human Movement Science, 2005;24,574–587.

[175] Noble JJ, Charles-Edwards GD, Keevil SF, Lewis AP, Gough M, Shortland AP. Intramuscular fat in ambulant young adults with bilateral spastic cerebral palsy. BMC Musculoskeletal Disorders, 2014;15: 236.

[176] Snider L, Korner-Bitensky N, Kammann C, Warner S, Saleh M. Horseback riding as therapy for children with cerebral palsy: Is there evidence of its effectiveness? Physical and Occupational Therapy in Pediatrics. 2007;27:5–23.

[177] Champagne D, Corriveau H, Dugas C. Effect of hippotherapy on motor proficiency and function in children with cerebral palsy who walk. Physical and Occupational Therapy in Pediatrics. 2016;1:1-13.

[178] Strauss, I. Hippotherapy: Neurophysiological therapy on the horse. Toronto, Ontario: Therapeutic Riding Association; 1995.

[179] Van Roon D, Steenbergen B, Meulenbroek RG. Trunk recruitment during spoon use in tetraparetic cerebral palsy. Experimental Brain Research. 2004;155:186–195.

[180] Wuang YP, Su CY. Reliability and responsiveness of the Bruininks–Oseretsky Test of Motor Proficiency—In children with intellectual disability. Research in Developmental Disabilities. 2009;30:847–855.

[181] Park ES, Rha DW, Shin JS, Kim S, Jung S. Effects of hippotherapy on gross motor function and functional performance of children with cerebral palsy. Yonsei Medical Journal. 2014;55:1736-1742. DOI: 10.3349/ymj.2014.55.6.1736.

[182] Kwon TG, Yi SH, Kim TW, Chang HJ, Kwon JY. Relationship between gross motor function and daily functional skill in children with cerebral palsy. Annals of Rehabilitation Medicine. 2013;37:41-49.

[183] Casady RL, Nichols-Larsen DS. The effect of hippotherapy on ten children with cerebral palsy. Pediatric Physical Therapy. 2004;16:165-172.

Chapter 4

ICF-CY-Based Physiotherapy Management in Children with Cerebral Palsy

Özge Çankaya and Kübra Seyhan

Additional information is available at the end of the chapter

http://dx.doi.org/10.5772/64255

Abstract

The immature brain damage causes cerebral palsy (CP) in children, and these children have many disorders of movement and posture development, often accompanied by disturbances of sensation, perception, cognition, communication, and behavior and by epilepsy and secondary musculoskeletal problems. According to the children and youth version of the WHO's classification as *International Classification of* Functioning, *Disability* and *Health*—child and youth (ICF-CY), function can be classified, measured, and influenced in several dimensions. In the treatment of CP, various approaches used are based on different theories of motor learning. Commonly used approaches in the treatment of children with CP are as follows: (1) neurodevelopmental therapy, (2) goal-directed therapy, (3) constraint-induced movement therapy, (4) bimanual intensive manual therapy, (5) treadmill training, (6) muscle strength training, (7) virtual reality, (8) aquatherapy, (9) hippotherapy, (10) family education and home-based treatment.

Keywords: cerebral palsy, ICF-CY, physiotherapy, motor learning

1. Introduction

Cerebral palsy (CP) is a permanent, nonprogressive disorder that occurred in the developing fetus or infant brain, causing deformity in posture and movement development and activity limitation [1, 2].

Movement deformity in CP is characterized clinically with the positive and negative signs of the upper motor neuron syndrome. The positive findings are abnormal phenomena, which occur due to inhibition deficiency emerging in clinical examination frequently. The positive findings are spasticity, dyskinesia, hyperreflexia, delayed developmental reactions, and secondary muscle-skeletal malformations. The negative findings are disability reflecting deficiency or the absence of development of sensory-motor control mechanisms, decrease in movement coordination, and weak balance and walking ability [3–5].

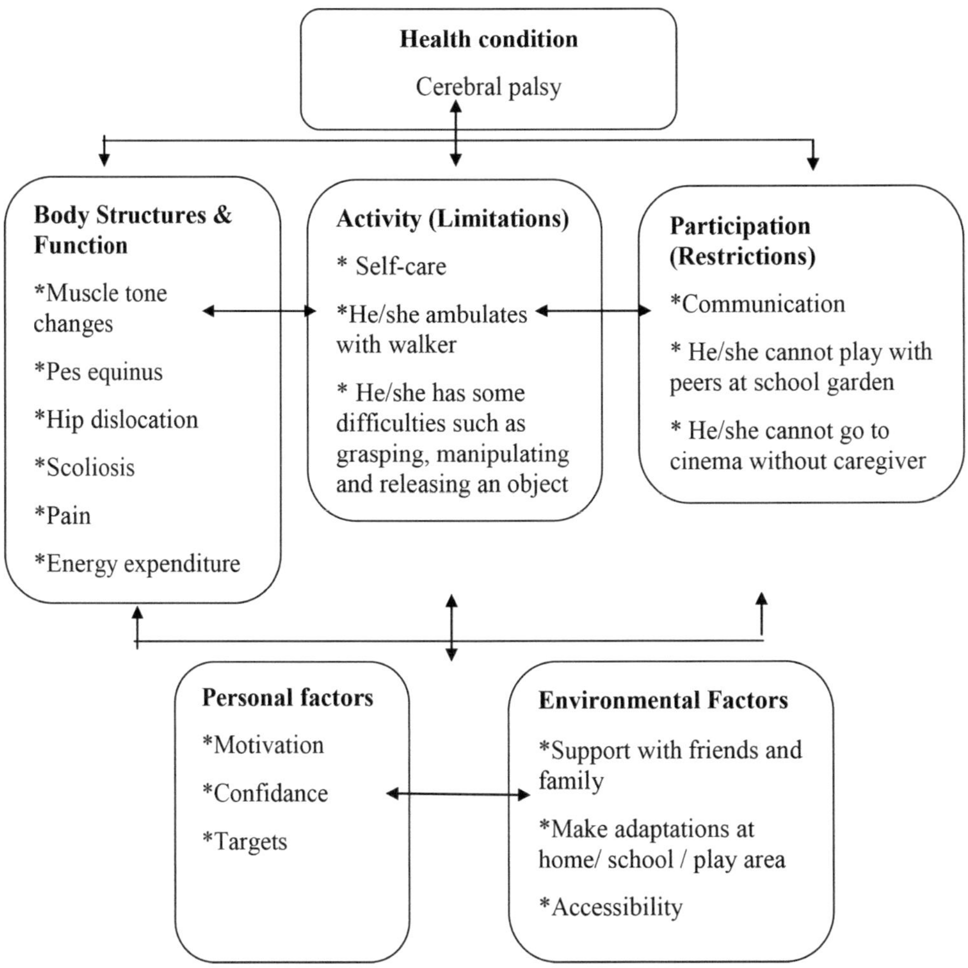

Table 1. ICF-CY three for cerebral palsy.

The World Health Organization's (WHO's) *International Classification of Functioning, Disability, and Health* (ICF), including its *Children and Youth* version (CY), established specifically to determine health state of children and youngsters and consisting of 1685 categories, is a considerably wide-scale coding system [6]. ICF-CY is a biopsychosocial model that emphasizes human functioning (body functions and structures, activities, and participation) as a result of the interaction between health conditions (diseases or diagnoses) and contextual factors [classified and coded as environmental (e) and personal factors] [6]. General definitions used in ICF-CY are as follows:

- Body functions are physiologic functions of body systems.
- Body structures are anatomic parts such as organs and limbs of the body.
- Impairment is the problems and deviations in body structures and functions and losses of functions.
- Activity is doing a movement or task by the individual.
- Participation is to be within life.
- Activity limitation is the difficulty during activities in the life of the individual.
- Restriction in participation is the problems that an individual may encounter in life.
- Environmental factors make up the physical, social, and mental factors in the environment of the individual [6].

In recent years, ICF-CY is a guide used prevalently in both the evaluation of children and the determination of a treatment program. The impairments observed in CP according to ICF-CY are outlined in **Table 1**. The therapeutic approaches used in CP treatment on the base of ICF-CY are summarized above.

2. Neuro-developmental therapy

Neuro-developmental therapy (NDT) or Bobath therapy is one of the prevalently used therapeutic approaches established by Berta and Karel Bobath in 1940s [7]. Developments in Bobath approach have continued since 1940 until today and now are a "living concept" rather than a technique [8]. This concept consists of specific theories improved by experiences, and these theories have been developed until today by preserving their dynamics along with various changes [9]. Recently, Bobath concept is congruent with the ICF-CY, acknowledging the entirety of human functioning in all spheres of life, as well as the individual nature of each problems. Activity limitations are regarded as the outcome of a complex relationship between the individual's health condition, personal factors, and the external factors of the environmental circumstances in which the individual lives. The structure provided by the ICF-CY has moved the focus of clinicians beyond interventions that are only impairments directed toward enabling the individual to overcome activity and participation restrictions. Participation restrictions are identified in consultation with the individual, the family, and relevant caregivers. The functional goals that are set are those that are relevant and achievable for the individual [10].

The concept comprises three fundamental rules as facilitation, communication, and stimulation to ensure normal postural experiences, reduce motor sensory impairments, and to improve functional independency level in children with CP. Handling techniques that control various sensory inputs are used, to regulate abnormal tonus, reflexes, and movement patterns and at the same time to facilitate muscle tonus, balance, and normal movement patterns [11, 12]. Functions that cannot be carried out by children due to spasticity or muscle fluctuation are determined and personal target analysis is made. Tonus regulation is ensured by positioning. Active movements are revealed by stimulations improving sensorimotor activity [10, 13]. Numerous modifications can be made in treatment since NDT is a "living concept."

The Bobath concept strives toward a 24-h interdisciplinary management approach. When the individual, family, all professionals, and other caregivers have insight into the problems and work together for the same goals, these goals are usually accomplished. Motivation and the therapeutic relationship between the clinician, the patient, and their family and/or caregivers are recognized as essential aspects for successful rehabilitation. The holistic approach to intervention is integral to the Bobath concept. The Bobath concept is an interactive problem-solving approach. Reassessment is ongoing with attention to individual goals, development of working hypotheses, treatment plans, and relevant objective measures to evaluate interventions. Intervention strategies are unique to the individual [10].

When the researches in the literature are considered, Weindling et al. [14] compared the NDT with standard care applications in their study conducted on 87 infants and showed that there were similar results in both groups. Mayo et al. [15] applied NDT to 17 infants diagnosed with CP one time a week, and the other 12 infants one time a month for 6 months. In conclusion, it was found that intensive NDT application showed better motor development. Palmer et al. [16] applied an "infant stimulation program" consisting of family-based motor, sense, language, and cognitive activities for a year to spastic infants with CP in the age range of 12 to 19 months old. Franki et al. showed in their systematic review that NDT's effects were arranged on their evidence levels according to ICF, and NDT is a method for improving gross motor function level, and activity, and participation level. It was reported that functionality was ensured by the regulation of muscle tonus and muscle length enabled by NDT [13].

Although NDT is the most prevalently used treatment by physiotherapists in Northern America, there is not sufficient evidence to support its effects [17, 18]. It is very difficult to compare it with other applications because of the modifications made in the original method generally [19].

Summary

Neuro-developmental therapy is summarized as follows:

- NDT is an interactive problem-solving approach.
- NDT strives toward a 24-h interdisciplinary management approach.
- NDT improves motor performance, especially gross motor skill, postural control, and stability.
- NDT can be effective in each parameter of ICF-CY.

3. Goal-directed therapy

Goal-directed therapy (GDT) consists of recovery based on brain plasticity after brain lesion depending on motor learning, motor control, biomechanics, muscle physiology, and activity. It is used recently in the pediatric rehabilitation field frequently. In this application, functional activity is organized according to the behavioral goals instead of isolated reflexes or motor patterns according to the theory of dynamic system of motor control. The therapists ensure active participation of children and attempt to change environmental limitations by various means in order to assist the solution of motor deficit in the central nervous system (CNS) [20].

One of the major problems in CP is the abnormal programming of movement. GDT is an application aiming smooth programming of movement according to motor learning principles. According to the assessment of ICF-CY, ensuring of maximum independency and functionality of children is aimed by the goals determined for activity limitation and participation constraint [21]. The therapy focuses on active participation to improve functional independency and performance instead of elimination of deficits [22].

In the literature, it is reported that very effective gain can be achieved in personal functional goals and gross motor function by the goal arrangements specific to person as a result of the goal-oriented and functional applications. Numerous individual goals are defined according to the activity level. In short term, especially measurable, specific therapy goals are effective in the motivation of therapists, family, and children [23]. It was shown that there was significant change in the participation level of children with CP by goal-oriented training [24]. The families expressed that they were satisfied with the therapy and goal-determination process and this situation created positive effect on the surrounding of the children [25].

Summary

Goal-directed therapy is summarized as follows:

- GDT is applied according to motor-learning principle.
- The goals must be specific to individuals and measurable.
- Goal-oriented active participation and environmental arrangement is crucial.
- GDT is effective in each level of ICF-CY.

4. Constraint-induced movement therapy

Constraint-induced movement therapy (CIMT) is a rehabilitation technique developed by Edward Taub [26] supporting "repetitive" use of the upper limbs in hemiparetic patients. Initial studies were conducted on monkeys who were made to develop somatosensorial deafferentation by preventing somatic sensory modulation in the upper limbs. Following somatosensorial deafferentation, "learned nonuse" idea was introduced when the monkeys were not able to use their arms effected in the free setting. CIMT approach was initially used in adult hemiparetic patients and it is limited healthy upper limbs or slightly affected upper limbs for breaking "learned nonuse" pattern [27]. The following three key components are used to improve usage of the affected upper limbs in CIMT:

- Constraining healthy upper limb movements
- Intense practice
- Shaping of behavior

The application showed successful results in adults, and subsequently, it was used in children with hemiparetic CP as well. As different from adults, CIMT is applied in the framework of motor learning rules in the earliest term in hemiplegic children because the right movement was never learned [28]. Children with hemiplegic CP may have sensorial problems as well such as asterognosis with the effection of the areas related with the pyrimidal system, talamocortical ways, somatosensorial areas, and sensorial integration [29]. The purpose of CIMT approach is to prevent the ignorance of the affected side, learned nonuse, and poor plasticity. It is desired in the studies in general that children's cognitive level is good, 20° of extension in the effect side wrist is achieved, and there is the skill to be able to release an object from their hands [28, 30]. According to ICF-CY, CIMT promotes functional changes that permit children with hemiplegic CP to increase their participation in various tasks outside of therapy and by improving the ability to perform upper limb tasks in a lasting way. Intervention in a natural setting accounts for the importance of the individual's environment and might facilitate the transfer of any learned skills into daily functioning.

The original program consists of a 6-h training a day for 3 weeks for low-function patients [31]. Today, the application has been modified in various forms according to the constraint period, materials used for constraint purpose, and application setting. Constraint form of the healthy limb in children can be ensured by casts, braces, orthesis, slings, or gloves [28]. Constraint duration varies from 30 min to 6 h according to the children's age and adaptation. CIMT approach can be applied as a daily therapy session, weekly camp model, or house-based therapy session [32]. An enriched environment and active motor training are crucial again [33]. CIMT effectiveness was shown at the age range of 7 months and 30 years old; however, there is no evidence yet for the effectiveness of early physiotherapy. There was no difference found in the developments following CIMT application of the same intensity in children of 4–8 years of old and 9–13 years of old [28]. By the daily camp model of Thompson et al., modified CIMP was applied to six children with hemiparetic CP and progress was achieved in hand skills, personal care, and social functions of the children [34]. Chen et al. reported better motor control changes induced by a home-based CIMT program compared with a dose-matched clinic-based traditional therapy, which included neuro-developmental treatment techniques and unilateral and bilateral activity-oriented training [35]. A randomized controlled trial investigated the same modified regimen of CIMT in two groups. The only differences arose from the randomization to either the home-based therapeutic environment, where the children had the opportunity to engage in real-life conditions using their own toys, or the clinic-based environment. The findings revealed greater improvements in the home-based group [36].

Summary

CIMT is summarized as follows:

- Three key components of CIMT are the constraint of healthy hand movement, intense practice, and behavior shaping.
- CIMT application may be modified according to age, motivation of child, duration of exercise, environmental setting, and constraint devices.
- CIMT is effective on all parameters of the ICF-CY.

5. Bimanual intensive manual therapy

One of the task-oriented therapies in children with hemiparetic CP is intense bimanual therapy (BIMT). Bimanual activities are difficult for hemiplegic children [37]. In bimanual activities, whereas one of the hands is stabilized normally, the dominant hand is engaged in more active procedures, and the children with hemiplegic CP develop compensatory single hand strategies (e.g., they achieve stabilization of an object by using their mouths and knees) by using other parts of the body because they cannot use their affected hand sufficiently for support [29]. This application is an approach used according to motor learning principles in children with hemiplegic CP. The purpose is to improve usage quality and characteristics bimanually. Furthermore, performance is more important. Both hands are used actively [38]. Active fine-gross motor movements according to the age and functional level of children are determined. First, active movements are shown with the healthy limb and the activities are repeated with the affected side. Difficulty and speed of the task is graded [39]. The upper extremity, which is used as a stabilizator at the beginning, is moved for more difficult manipulative skills over time. In the study of Gordon et al. comparing BIMT and CIMT applications, CIMT was found to be more effective in solving the impairment, and BIMT was found to be more effective in bimanual motor coordination and planning. Moreover, it was reported that a 90-h BIMT application was more effective in comparison to a 60-h application. Studies on the therapy frequencies are still ongoing [37].

Summary

BIMT is summarized as follows:

- BIMT aims the quality bilateral upper extremity use.
- It is applied according to motor learning principles.
- It is more motivating and child-friendly because it is not a constraining material.

6. Treadmill training

Treadmill training is a method encompassing motor learning and motor control theories and used for improving postural control in children because it is based on repetition and practice

[40]. Walking limitations are faced frequently in CP. Reduced walking speed and endurance are the two fundamental problems [41]. Walking is with rhytmic steps and repeating patterns in treadmill training, and this improves harmonization between agonist and antagonist muscles and ensures the development of dynamic and static balance. The conducted studies illustrated that positive progress was achieved in gross motor function and gaiting with the treadmill training [40, 42].

In a systematic review conducted by Willoughby et al, the effects of treadmill training are as follows:

- *Effects on gross motor function*: Significant improvement was achieved in the gross motor function measure (GMFM)'s D (standing) and E (walking, running, jumping) and total score sections.
- *Efects on body structure and function*: Energy spent during walking was assessed and significant change in energy expenditure index (EEI) was observed. There was no significant change observed as a result of the evaluation of muscle tonus and selective motor control.
- *Effects on social participation*: The effects on social participation in children with CP have not been evaluated in any of the studies.
- *Adverse event*: Treadmill training was tolerated by all participants and there was no unexpected situation faced. There was no injury during or after the training due to any muscle spasm and joint ache or falling [43].

Treadmill training can be used in children with CP at any level of GMFCS. Based on the functional level of children, speed (range 0.25–5 km/h or as fast as possible), training period (and duration (10–30 min) and support amount provided to the children (Body weight support treadmill training (BWSTT) and partial body-weight support treadmill training (PBWSTT)) can change [44].

Body-weight support treadmill training (BWSTT) ensures stepping, endurance, and strengthening training in adults by reducing body weight. It is used less frequently in children. Following the declaration of the effects of early gaiting training in children with CP by Richard et al in 1997 [45], studies using BWSTT in children with CP have increased. It was reported that BWSTT could ensure positive improvement in gross motor function and walking speed; however, further randomized controlled studies were needed [46].

Partial body-weight support treadmill training (PBWSTT) allows the therapist systematically to train patients to walk on a treadmill at increasing speeds with increasing weight bearing, and simulating what will be necessary for household or community ambulation for GMFCS level IV and V children. PBWSTT intervention is also potentially attractive as it may address gait limitations more effectively, because it allows gait to be addressed at multiple levels of ICF-CY. Interest in PBWSTT for children with CP is rapidly increasing. Evidence to support treatment intervention in children with CP should be carefully explored by clinicians before they add it to their treatment repertoires.

In the literature, it was reported that improvement could be achieved in self-selected walking speed and gross motor function by PBWSTT in children with CP [47, 48].

Summary

Treadmill training is summarized as follows:

- Treadmill training is appropriate for children in any GMFCS levels.
- The speed is generally 0.25–5 km/h and duration is 10–30 min.
- It has positive effects on body structure and function in comparison to ICF-CY.

7. Muscle strength training

Muscular weakness presents a serious problem for children with CP [49]. In the past, strengthening training was avoided with the notion that it would increase spasticity and reduce range of motion (ROM) and cause gaiting problems in children with CP. It was shown in the conducted systematic reviews that strengthening training is effective in muscle strengthening without any negative effect [50]. Resistive training improves muscular force and muscular volume, and this force can be transferred to the functional development [2, 51]. Progressive resistance exercise (PRE) is a strengthening training method where intensity is increased over time. It stimulates strength gain more in comparison to normal development and growth. Fundamental principles of PRE can complete small repetitions with an effective resistance without the creation of exhaustion in a set. According to the National Strength and Conditioning Association (NSCA), the principles of the strengthening training in youngsters are outlined as follows:

- Ensuring quality training and supervision.
- Make sure that the exercise setting is safe and free of danger.
- Start to each exercise session with a 5–10 min dynamic warming period.
- Start with rather light loads and focus on the right exercise technique always.
- Do the various upper and lower extremity strengthening exercises with 6–15 repetition and as 1–3 sets.
- It must consist of special exercises to strengthen abdominal and back regions.
- Focus on the development of symmetrical muscles around the joints and on appropriate muscular balance.
- Apply various upper and lower extremities force exercises with 3–6 repetitions and as 1–3 sets.
- Advance in the training program based on need, goal, and skills.
- Increase the resistance gradually (5–10%) as the force increases.
- Cool down with calistenic and static stretch exercises.
- Listen to personal needs and anxieties in each session.

- Start the endurance training 2–3 times a week in nonconsecutive days.
- Use personal loading to observe the progress.
- Keep the program fresh and make systematic changes in the training program.
- Make the performance suitable and compose with healthy nutrition, adequate hydration, and proper sleep.
- Support and encouragement by the family and trainer will help increase in interest [52].

Although the duration and arrangement of PRE training in children with CP is still contradictive, the selection of candidate and exercise contributes to the improvement of daily functions in various degrees including gross motor function and gait quality. It was illustrated that PRE created muscular force without generating harmful effects, such as hypertonia, and improved children's skills [53].

In the review of Verschuren et al, it was reported that before starting strengthening exercises in children with CP, there must be an exercise "adaption period" for 2–4 weeks, two times a week, and for this, starting with low dose (with short duration, less intense, consisting of a single joint) exercises than the duration and intensity of exercises are increased as the adaptation of the children improves and can be started multiple joints exercises.

The strengthening training suggested for children with CP is as follows:

- *Frequency*: 2–4 times a week in nonconsecutive days
- *Intensity:* in 50–85% of maximum repetition, 6–15 repeats, 1–3 sets
- *Duration:* the period of a special training has not been defined for an effect. The training period must be at least in consecutive 12–16 weeks.
- *Type:* initially single joint, machine-based exercises must be started and then, multijoint endurance exercises must follow with the machines plus free weight (closed kinetic chain). Single-joint endurance training at the beginning of the training may be more effective for very weak muscles in children [54].

In the pilot study of Blundell et al conducted on a small group of children with CP at the ages of 4–8 years old, 47% force increase was achieved in the children with PRE training applied by using gymnastics equipments, including treadmill and leg press as a group training 2 days a week for 4 weeks, and this effect continued for 8 weeks following the application [55].

In the study of Ault et al, low-dose community-based strengthening training was applied in children with CP, and at the end of the study, in addition to the functional force activities, significant gain was achieved in protective postural adjustment, static stability limit, and dynamic balance. It was indicated that low-dose exercises can be effective as well without a need for expensive equipment [53].

As a result of the strengthening training of Bania et al applied for 12 weeks 2 days a week accompanied with physiotherapists in sports hall in children with bilateral spastic CP, it was reported that force increase was achieved in the lower extremity muscles; however, there was

http://dx.doi.org/10.5772/64255

no significant change in daily physical activity. Whereas improvement was achieved in body functions in the scope of ICF-CY, activity, and participation was not affected [56]. In the systematic review of Franki et al, the strengthening training showed changes in body structure and functions such as decrease in energy consumption, increase in muscle volume, improvement in body image perception in comparison to ICF-CY. An increase in gait and gross motor function and development in activity was reported. There was no effect of strengthening training on participation found in the articles [44].

In a review, the effect of the upper extremity strengthening training in children with CP, it was indicated that there was no adequate randomized controlled studies, in addition to the strengthening training, goal-oriented therapy, electric stimulation, and botulinum toxin applications were conducted. According to NSCA's criteria, resistance exercises were suggested for at least 12 weeks three times a week, with 8–15 repetition. The effect on activity and participation was not evaluated in any of the studies [57].

Summary

Muscle strength training is summarized as follows:

- The strengthening training in children with CP improves the force and muscle volume without any adverse effect.
- PRE training is applied at least 3 days a week with 8–12 repetition, 1–3 sets and for 8–20 weeks for each muscle.
- The muscle force achieved by PRE training must be transferred to functional activities.

8. Virtual reality

Virtual reality (VR) systems ensure opportunity for children with CP to do performance activities that they cannot do in his/her natural environment by establishing an interactive and motivating setting. These systems provide feedback to the player in virtual world and the child can observe their own movements. VR improves motor skills with repetitive practices oriented to the goal in children with CP due to its characteristics, including task separation between the real world and virtual environment, with flexible therapy parameters specific to the person, visual and audial feedback, social game equality during game, neuroplastic changes, problem solving in different virtual situations, motivation of the children in game selection and completion, and undertaking a supportive role in verbal encouragement and feedback. All of these parameters are required for motor learning and improvement of motor skills [58, 59]. Modifications can be made in exercise dose (duration, frequency, intensity).

Movement-based interactive video games (IVO): Nintendo Wii and Microsoft's Kinect movement sensors are the new treatment methods for children with CP. They improve arm movements, functional status, daily life activities, and balance of children [60–62]. In the study of Luna Oliva et al [63], balance and daily life activities of children with CP who were treated for 8 weeks with Xbox 360 Kinect ™ (Microsoft) improved. Positive developments were determined following therapy in gross motor functions, balance, gait speed, running and jumping, daily life activities, and fine motor skills of children. Although IVO is used as a treatment method in many studies, it can also be used as an evaluation method. Kinect 360 Xbox sensor provides information about the speed, acceleration, and distance of movement [63]. In the study of Jelsma et al. conducted on children with hemiparetic cerebrals palsy, it was revealed that Nintendo Wii Fit game is effective in balance training [64].

It was reported that virtual reality systems were effective and used in the fields including upper limb (quality of the movement, active movement control and coordination of upper limb motor performance), lower limb (ankle kinematics, gait, functional performance), postural control (active control of pelvis and trunk, increased balance and selective control), and physical-cardiovascular fitness (great potential to promote increased physical activity and enhanced cardiovascular fitness) [65].

In the systematic review of Glegg et al, it was stated that there were scarce randomized controlled studies showing the effect of VR systems. The studies in the scope of ICF-CY showed that they generally evaluated functional balance and mobility, upper limbs, cognition, fitness, daily life activities, and living skills at home and in society and that VR systems were effective on body functions, activity, and participation.

Summary

Virtual reality is summarized as follows:

- VR systems encourage the child with funny and enjoyable play settings and increase child's motivation.
- The interactive games support motor learning and cortical plasticity.
- VR presents an opportunity to promote physical fitness and decrease sedentary behavior.

9. Aquatherapy

Aquatic exercises are performed within water by benefiting from various characteristics of water. Aquatherapy (AT) is an intervention applied with the assistance of an experienced therapist to benefit from mechanical characteristics of water. It is an application made of various activities selected specifically according to the problem of the participant and determined according to task-oriented motor learning principles [66, 67]. Although the term "aquatherapy" is used prevalently, many different terms are used as well including aquatic exercise therapy, aquatic rehabilitation, pool therapy, and hydrotherapy [68–70].

Children with CP can easily do many activities in water requiring movement control against gravity such as walking that they cannot do on land owing to physical and mechanical characteristics of water. Water gives a chance to the children to feel independent and improves their self-confidence and self-respect [71]. Movements within water are displayed with more control and slowly, and therefore, they ensure realization of postural reactions and required adjustments [72]. They can do the abnormally displayed movement patterns on land more smoothly in water. Mental awareness and focusing enhances in children who receive intense sense input with thermoregulation, waves, turbulence, viscosity, stretching force, and texture of water. Approaches in water can also be applied as a group activity in children whose motor functions and mental levels are in harmony with each other [73]. Doing activities in an entertaining and social setting for children also supports participation [74]. In the study of Brunton et al conducted on children with CP, exercise and activity participations of children according to their gross motor function levels (GMFCS I-V) were investigated. It was reported as a result of the study that children with good motor function level (I–III) preferred first walking activity and then swimming activity; children with low level (IV–V) preferred walking activity first [75]). In the scope of ICF-CY, it is crucial to enhance activity and participation of children with neuromotor problems, and in this respect, water provides a suitable setting [76]. When the studies in the literature are considered, the treatment frequency and duration is 20–40 min a day for 2–5 days a week and at least 14–16 weeks in total [77]. A lifting system within pool can be constructed for participants whose function level is low.

Aquatherapy is concerned with all parameters under ICF-CY frame. Halliwick technique is an efficient approach for children who cannot do activities due to insufficiencies in their body structure and functions and whose social participation is constrained [66, 77]. This approach, requiring active participation, ensures the children to do many processes that they cannot do on land, within water, and receiving a group training along with children at their own motor function level increases their social participation [73, 78]. High motivation of children within water, which is an entertaining environment, affects their motor-learning process [70, 79]. Furthermore, satisfaction of the children and families provides positive feedbacks as personal and environmental factors [80]. Dimitrijevic investigated the effect of techniques in water on gross motor function and skills in water in children with CP. A therapy protocol was applied made up of 10-min warm up, 40-min swimming, and 5-min game activities for 6 weeks (55 min/2 sessions/week) to the children. Motor function skills improved significantly in water and on land in AT group [81]. Getz et al. examined the effect of AT on motor performance and metabolic consumption during walking in children with early-stage spastic diplegic CP. It was observed that AT reduced metabolic consumption during walking at the end of a 16-week program. While oxygen consumption value was conserved, walking speed increased during submaximal exercise [82]. Gorter evaluated aquatic exercise programs in the scope of ICF-CY in a review conducted on adolescent children with CP. It was reported that AT participation was constrained in children who are influenced strongly by personal and environmental factors (barriers) including fear and transportation problems. Progress was observed in walking and running activities, balance skills, energy consumption indexes, muscular forces, and performance tests [83].

Summary

Aquatherapy is summarized as follows:

- Thermoregulation, waves, turbulence, viscosity, lifting force, and water texture is used as therapeutics in AT.

- AT is related with all parameters under the ICF-CY.
- The frequency of treatment is 20–40 min/daily, 2–5 day/week and between 14–16 weeks.

10. Hippotherapy

Hippotherapy (HT) is an approach used highly by physiotherapy, occupational therapy, and speech therapists to ensure motor and sensorial stimulus in children who need therapy. Typical characteristics are benefited including rhythmic movements and body heat of horse for the therapy purpose [84]. In therapeutic horse riding, the purpose is based on teaching of horse riding and control skills, and HT is completely a treatment strategy and is used in neuro-developmental disorders including cerebral palsy and autism and in the treatment of adult patients who have neurologic disorder [85]. HT practitioner is called hippotherapist. Within HT sessions, there must be a therapeutic horse, patient, "puller" directing the horse, "side walker" responsible for patient safety, and a hippotherapist responsible for execution of the session with all of these people [86]. HT can continue for 30 min–1 h a day, 1–2 sessions a week, and for 12–18 weeks in total [87].

According to body structure and function dimension of ICF-CY, it decreased muscle tone and improved trunk and pelvic posture and stability and child behavior. On activities, significant improvements on upper and lower limb gross motor function was reported [44, 88].

Summary

HT is summarized as follows:

- HT can be used as an addition to all treatments to develop posture and postural control.
- The intensity of treatment is approximately 30 min–1 h/day, duration of HT is 1–2 day/week during 12–18 weeks.

11. Family education and home-based treatment

Family is at the center of treatment in all treatment methods for children with CP. In addition to have the children do home exercises who spend large portion of the day within home setting, it is crucial that children are observed during life activities, including personal care, mobility and sleep, and appropriate adaptations, are provided to protect their body structures, and functionality is continued [89].

Family education principles acknowledge that families are different and unique, and optimal child functioning occurs within a supportive family and community context and that parents know their children best with the therapist viewed as a collaborator, not as an expert. Goals of treatment are identified collaboratively with input from the family, child, and therapist. There is evidence to indicate that family education leads to improved outcomes for children

http://dx.doi.org/10.5772/64255

and families as well as greater satisfaction for families leading to increased adherence to treatment recommendations and to improved well-being and fewer parental feelings of distress and depression [90].

The Coping with and Caring for Infants with Special Needs (COPCA) Program is a treatment method aiming activity and participation in children with CP by teaching home exercises to families and routine monitoring. The center of COPCA is family. Therefore, family autonomy, family responsibility, and family-specific parenthood are the fundamental components of COPCA. Family autonomy shows the criteria of family for living quality. Family responsibility reflects the selections and decisions of family about child care and the interaction of health professionals. Family-specific parenthood illustrates the child training form of caregiver for the child to have responsibility and be independent. The purpose of COPCA program is to encourage families to solve daily care problems that are observed naturally during parenthood by using their own capacity. “Coaching” is used to reach this goal. Coaching is the fundamental strategy of COPCA. The coaches (physiotherapists) do not tell the families what they can do or what they should do but they help families discover applications that can be carried out. Physiotherapists listen to families, make observations and suggestions, and inform and support them. Families are the persons who have major responsibility to make decisions about the child care and treatment with the help of the physiotherapist.

In the study of Dirks et al, it was illustrated that the infants showed development in supine, prone, and sitting positions according to the results of the evaluations performed in month 4 and 6 in risky infants who were treated by using COPCA method. In addition to the progress in the development of the children, there were positive developments in activity in the scope of ICF-CY [91].

The following conditions must be considered for a home program to be effective:

- Parents must be in collaboration and know the child and child's home setting well.
- Children and families must determine which work they want to do in home setting and select a goal accordingly.
- Selection of home program among evidence-based applications, selection of the purposes according to family life, and changing them according to the preferences of children
- Providing regular support to the families to define the development of the children and to determine the things to be added to the program
- Evaluation of the results together.

Summary

Family education and home-based treatment is summarized as follows:

- Family is in the center of the treatment.
- Family education leads to improved outcomes for children and families as well as greater satisfaction for families leading to increased adherence to all kinds of therapeutic treatments.
- Family should be supported by physiotherapists for the application of the home program.

Author details

Özge Çankaya* and Kübra Seyhan

*Address all correspondence to: ozgemuezzinoglu@gmail.com

Department of Physiotherapy and Rehabilitation, Faculty of Health Sciences, Hacetepe University, Ankara, Turkey

References

[1] Bax M, Goldstein M, Rosenbaum P, Leviton A, Paneth N, Dan B, et al. Proposed definition and classification of cerebral palsy, April 2005. Developmental Medicine & Child Neurology. 2005;47(08):571–6.

[2] Stark C, Nikopoulou-Smyrni P, Stabrey A, Semler O, Schoenau E. Effect of a new physiotherapy concept on bone mineral density, muscle force and gross motor function in children with bilateral cerebral palsy. 2010.

[3] Pandyan AD, Gregoric M, Barnes MP, Wood D, Wijck Fv, Burridge J, et al. Spasticity: clinical perceptions, neurological realities and meaningful measurement. Disability and Rehabilitation. 2005;27(1–2):2–6.

[4] Goldstein EM. Spasticity management: an overview. Journal of Child Neurology. 2001;16(1):16–23.

[5] Rosenbaum P, Paneth N, Leviton A, Goldstein M, Bax M, Damiano D, et al. A report: the definition and classification of cerebral palsy April 2006. Developmental Medicine & Child Neurology Supplement. 2007;109(suppl 109):8–14.

[6] World Health Organization. International classification of functioning, disability, and health: children & youth version: ICF-CY: World Health Organization; 2007.

[7] Bobath B. A neuro-developmental treatment of cerebral palsy. Physiotherapy. 1963;49:242.

[8] Bobath K. A neurophysiological basis for the treatment of cerebral palsy: Cambridge University Press; 1991.

[9] Türker D, Korkem D, Özal C, Günel MK, Karahan S. The effects of neuro-developmental (Bobath) therapy based goal directed therapy on gross motor function and functional status of children with cerebral palsy. International Journal of Therapies and Rehabilitation Research. 2015;4(4):9–20.

[10] Graham JV, Eustace C, Brock K, Swain E, Irwin-Carruthers S. The Bobath concept in contemporary clinical practice. Topics in Stroke Rehabilitation. 2009;16(1):57–68.

[11] Gunel MK. Rehabilitation of children with cerebral palsy from a physiotherapist's perspective. Acta Orthopaedica et Traumatologica Turcica. 2009;43(2):173–80.

[12] Howle JM. Neuro-developmental treatment approach: theoretical foundations and principles of clinical practice. NeuroDevelopmental Treatment; 2002.

[13] Molenaers G, Calders P, Vanderstraeten G, Himpens E. The evidence-base for conceptual approaches and additional therapies targeting lower limb function in children with cerebral palsy: a systematic review using the international classification of functioning, disability and health as a framework. Journal of Rehabilitation Medicine. 2012;44(5): 396–405.

[14] Weindling A, Hallam P, Gregg J, Klenka H, Rosenbloom L, Hutton J. A randomized controlled trial of early physiotherapy for high-risk infants. Acta Paediatrica. 1996;85(9):1107–11.

[15] Mayo NE. The effect of physical therapy for children with motor delay and cerebral palsy: a randomized clinical trial. American Journal of Physical Medicine & Rehabilitation. 1991;70(5):258–67.

[16] Palmer FB, Shapiro BK, Wachtel RC, Allen MC, Hiller JE, Harryman SE, et al. The effects of physical therapy on cerebral palsy. New England Journal of Medicine. 1988;318(13): 803–8.

[17] Dumas HM, O'Neil ME, Fragala MA. Expert consensus on physical therapist intervention after botulinum toxin A injection for children with cerebral palsy. Pediatric Physical Therapy. 2001;13(3):122–32.

[18] Saleh M, Korner-Bitensky N, Snider L, Malouin F, Mazer B, Kennedy E, et al. Actual vs. best practices for young children with cerebral palsy: a survey of paediatric occupational therapists and physical therapists in Quebec, Canada. Developmental Neurorehabilitation. 2008;11(1):60–80.

[19] Tyson S, Connell L, Busse M, Lennon S. What is Bobath? A survey of UK stroke physiotherapists' perceptions of the content of the Bobath concept to treat postural control and mobility problems after stroke. Disability and rehabilitation. 2009;31(6): 448–57.

[20] Smith LB, Thelen E. Development as a dynamic system. Trends in Cognitive Sciences. 2003;7(8):343–8.

[21] Law M, Darrah J, Pollock N, Rosenbaum P, Russell D, Walter SD, et al. Focus on Function–a randomized controlled trial comparing two rehabilitation interventions for young children with cerebral palsy. BMC Pediatrics. 2007;7(1):31.

[22] Palisano RJ, Snider LM, Orlin MN, editors. Recent advances in physical and occupational therapy for children with cerebral palsy. Seminars in Pediatric Neurology; 2004: Elsevier.

[23] Bower E, McLellan D, Amey J, Campbell M. A randomised controlled: trial of different intensities of physiotherapy and different goal-setting procedures in 44 children with cerebral palsy. Developmental Medicine & Child Neurology. 1996;38(3):226–37.

[24] Ketelaar M, Vermeer A, Hart Ht, van Petegem-van Beek E, Helders PJ. Effects of a functional therapy program on motor abilities of children with cerebral palsy. Physical Therapy. 2001;81(9):1534–45.

[25] Ahl LE, Johansson E, Granat T, Carlberg EB. Functional therapy for children with cerebral palsy: an ecological approach. Developmental Medicine & Child Neurology. 2005;47(9):613–9.

[26] Taub E, Crago JE, Uswatte G. Constraint-induced movement therapy: A new approach to treatment in physical rehabilitation. Rehabilitation Psychology. 1998;43(2):152.

[27] Taub E, Uswatte G, Pidikiti R. Constraint-Induced Movement Therapy: a new family of techniques with broad application to physical rehabilitation--a clinical review. Journal of Rehabilitation Research and Development. 1999;36(3):237.

[28] Gordon AM. To constrain or not to constrain, and other stories of intensive upper limb training for children with unilateral cerebral palsy. Developmental Medicine & Child Neurology. 2011;53(s4):56–61.

[29] Basu A, Eyre J. A plea for consideration of the less affected hand in therapeutic approaches to hemiplegia. Developmental Medicine & Child Neurology. 2012;54(4): 380–.

[30] Golomb MR, McDonald BC, Warden SJ, Yonkman J, Saykin AJ, Shirley B, et al. In-home virtual reality videogame telerehabilitation in adolescents with hemiplegic cerebral palsy. Archives of Physical Medicine and Rehabilitation. 2010;91(1):1–8. e1.

[31] Charles JR, Wolf SL, Schneider JA, Gordon AM. Efficacy of a child-friendly form of constraint-induced movement therapy in hemiplegic cerebral palsy: a randomized control trial. Developmental Medicine & Child Neurology. 2006;48(08):635–42.

[32] Gelkop N, Burshtein DG, Lahav A, Brezner A, Al-Oraibi S, Ferre CL, et al. Efficacy of constraint-induced movement therapy and bimanual training in children with hemiplegic cerebral palsy in an educational setting. Physical & Occupational Therapy in Pediatrics. 2015;35(1):24–39.

[33] Eliasson A-C, Sjöstrand L, Ek L, Krumlinde-Sundholm L, Tedroff K. Efficacy of baby-CIMT: study protocol for a randomised controlled trial on infants below age 12 months, with clinical signs of unilateral CP. BMC pediatrics. 2014;14(1):141.

[34] Thompson AM, Chow S, Vey C, Lloyd M. Constraint-induced movement therapy in children aged 5 to 9 years with cerebral palsy: a day camp model. Pediatric Physical Therapy. 2015;27(1):72–80.

[35] Chen H-c, Chen C-l, Kang L-j, Wu C-y, Chen F-c, Hong W-h. Improvement of upper limb motor control and function after home-based constraint induced therapy in

children with unilateral cerebral palsy: immediate and long-term effects. Archives of Physical Medicine and Rehabilitation. 2014;95(8):1423–32.

[36] Rostami HR, Malamiri RA. Effect of treatment environment on modified constraint-induced movement therapy results in children with spastic hemiplegic cerebral palsy: a randomized controlled trial. Disability and Rehabilitation. 2012;34(1):40–4.

[37] Gordon AM, Schneider JA, Chinnan A, Charles JR. Efficacy of a hand–arm bimanual intensive therapy (HABIT) in children with hemiplegic cerebral palsy: a randomized control trial. Developmental Medicine & Child Neurology. 2007;49(11):830–8.

[38] Dong VA-Q, Tung IH-H, Siu HW-Y, Fong KN-K. Studies comparing the efficacy of constraint-induced movement therapy and bimanual training in children with unilateral cerebral palsy: a systematic review. Developmental neurorehabilitation. 2013;16(2): 133–43.

[39] Aarts PB, Hartingsveldt M, Anderson PG, Tillaar I, Burg J, Geurts AC. The Pirate Group Intervention Protocol: Description and a Case Report of a Modified Constraint-induced Movement Therapy Combined with Bimanual Training for Young Children with Unilateral Spastic Cerebral Palsy. Occupational Therapy International. 2012;19(2):76–87.

[40] Hamah E. Effect of a new physical therapy concept on dynamic balance in children with spastic diplegic cerebral palsy. Egyptian Journal of Medical Human Genetics. 2015;16(1):77–83.

[41] Duffy C, Hill A, Cosgrove A, Carry I, Graham H. Energy consumption in children with spina bifida and cerebral palsy: a comparative study. Developmental Medicine & Child Neurology. 1996;38(3):238–43.

[42] Cho C, Hwang W, Hwang S, Chung Y. Treadmill Training with Virtual Reality Improves Gait, Balance, and Muscle Strength in Children with Cerebral Palsy. The Tohoku Journal of Experimental Medicine. 2016;238(3):213–8.

[43] Willoughby KL, Dodd KJ, Shields N. A systematic review of the effectiveness of treadmill training for children with cerebral palsy. Disability and Rehabilitation. 2009;31(24):1971–9.

[44] Franki I, Desloovere K, De Cat J, Feys H, Molenaers G, Calders P, et al. The evidence-base for basic physical therapy techniques targeting lower limb function in children with cerebral palsy: a systematic review using the International Classification of Functioning, Disability and Health as a conceptual framework. Journal of Rehabilitation Medicine. 2012;44(5):385–95.

[45] Richards CL, Malouin F, Dumas F, Marcoux S, Lepage C, Menier C. Early and intensive treadmill locomotor training for young children with cerebral palsy: a feasibility study. Pediatric Physical Therapy. 1997;9(4):158–65.

[46] Damiano DL, DeJong SL. A systematic review of the effectiveness of treadmill training and body weight support in pediatric rehabilitation. Journal of Neurologic Physical Therapy: JNPT. 2009;33(1):27.

[47] Chrysagis N, Skordilis EK, Stavrou N, Grammatopoulou E, Koutsouki D. The effect of treadmill training on gross motor function and walking speed in ambulatory adolescents with cerebral palsy: a randomized controlled trial. American Journal of Physical Medicine & Rehabilitation. 2012;91(9):747–60.

[48] Dodd KJ, Foley S. Partial body-weight-supported treadmill training can improve walking in children with cerebral palsy: a clinical controlled trial. Developmental Medicine & Child Neurology. 2007;49(2):101–5.

[49] Damiano DL, Dodd K, Taylor NF. Should we be testing and training muscle strength in cerebral palsy? Developmental Medicine & Child Neurology. 2002;44(01):68–72.

[50] Dodd KJ, Taylor NF, Graham HK. A randomized clinical trial of strength training in young people with cerebral palsy. Developmental Medicine & Child Neurology. 2003;45(10):652–7.

[51] Taylor NF, Dodd KJ, Damiano DL. Progressive resistance exercise in physical therapy: a summary of systematic reviews. Physical therapy. 2005;85(11):1208–23.

[52] Faigenbaum AD, Kraemer WJ, Blimkie CJ, Jeffreys I, Micheli LJ, Nitka M, et al. Youth resistance training: updated position statement paper from the national strength and conditioning association. The Journal of Strength & Conditioning Research. 2009;23:S60–79.

[53] Auld ML, Johnston LM. "Strong and steady": a community-based strength and balance exercise group for children with cerebral palsy. Disability and Rehabilitation. 2014;36(24):2065–71.

[54] Verschuren O, Peterson MD, Balemans AC, Hurvitz EA. Exercise and physical activity recommendations for people with cerebral palsy. Developmental Medicine & Child Neurology. 2016.

[55] Blundell S, Shepherd R, Dean C, Adams R, Cahill B. Functional strength training in cerebral palsy: a pilot study of a group circuit training class for children aged 4–8 years. Clinical Rehabilitation. 2003;17(1):48–57.

[56] Bania TA, Dodd KJ, Baker RJ, Graham HK, Taylor NF. The effects of progressive resistance training on daily physical activity in young people with cerebral palsy: a randomised controlled trial. Disability and Rehabilitation. 2015:1–7.

[57] Rameckers E, Janssen-Potten Y, Essers I, Smeets R. Efficacy of upper limb strengthening in children with cerebral palsy: a critical review. Research in Developmental Disabilities. 2015;36:87–101.

[58] Chen Y-p, Lee S-Y, Howard AM. Effect of virtual reality on upper limb function in children with cerebral palsy: a meta-analysis. Pediatric Physical Therapy. 2014;26(3): 289–300.

[59] Chiu H-C, Ada L, Lee H-M. Upper limb training using Wii Sports Resort™ for children with hemiplegic cerebral palsy: A randomized, single-blind trial. Clinical Rehabilitation. 2014;28(10):1015–24.

[60] Winkels DG, Kottink AI, Temmink RA, Nijlant JM, Buurke JH. Wii™-habilitation of upper limb function in children with cerebral palsy. An explorative study. Developmental neurorehabilitation. 2013;16(1):44–51.

[61] Tarakci D, Ozdincler AR, Tarakci E, Tutuncuoglu F, Ozmen M. Wii-based balance therapy to improve balance function of children with cerebral palsy: a pilot study. Journal of Physical Therapy Science. 2013;25(9):1123–7.

[62] Gordon C, Roopchand-Martin S, Gregg A. Potential of the Nintendo Wii™ as a rehabilitation tool for children with cerebral palsy in a developing country: a pilot study. Physiotherapy. 2012;98(3):238–42.

[63] Luna-Oliva L, Ortiz-Gutiérrez R, Cano-de la Cuerda R, Piédrola RM, Alguacil-Diego I, Sánchez-Camarero C. Evaluation of the use of a virtual reality video-game system as a supplement for rehabilitation of children with cerebral palsy. In: Converging Clinical and Engineering Research on Neurorehabilitation: Springer; 2013. pp. 873–7.

[64] Jelsma J, Pronk M, Ferguson G, Jelsma-Smit D. The effect of the Nintendo Wii Fit on balance control and gross motor function of children with spastic hemiplegic cerebral palsy. Developmental Neurorehabilitation. 2013;16(1):27–37.

[65] Kerem M, Kaya O, Ozal C, Turker D. Virtual reality in rehabilitation of children with cerebral palsy. 2014.

[66] Lambeck J, Gamper U. The halliwick concept. In: Comprehensive Aquatic Therapy. 3rd ed. Pullman, WA: Washington State University Publishing. 2011.

[67] Tripp F, Krakow K. Effects of an aquatic therapy approach (Halliwick-Therapy) on functional mobility in subacute stroke patients: a randomized controlled trial. Clinical Rehabilitation. 2014;28(5):432–9.

[68] Kelly M, Darrah J. Aquatic exercise for children with cerebral palsy. Developmental Medicine & Child Neurology. 2005;47(12):838–42.

[69] Verhagen AP, Cardoso JR, Bierma-Zeinstra SM. Aquatic exercise & balneotherapy in musculoskeletal conditions. Best Practice & Research Clinical Rheumatology. 2012;26(3):335–43.

[70] Getz M, Hutzler Y, Vermeer A. Effects of aquatic interventions in children with neuromotor impairments: a systematic review of the literature. Clinical Rehabilitation. 2006;20(11):927–36.

[71] Dumas H, Francesconi S. Aquatic therapy in pediatrics: annotated bibliography. Physical & Occupational Therapy in Pediatrics. 2001;20(4):63–78.

[72] Thein-Nissenbaum JM. Aquatic rehabilitation. Physical Rehabilitation of the Injured Athlete. 2011:295–314.

[73] Fragala-Pinkham M, Haley SM, O'Neil ME. Group aquatic aerobic exercise for children with disabilities. Developmental Medicine & Child Neurology. 2008;50(11):822–7.

[74] Takken T, Helders P. Description of Exercise Participation of Adolescents With Cerebral Palsy Across a 4-Year Period. Pediatric Physical Therapy. 2010;22(2):188.

[75] Brunton LK, Bartlett DJ. Description of exercise participation of adolescents with cerebral palsy across a 4-year period. Pediatric Physical Therapy. 2010;22(2):180–7.

[76] Schiariti V, Klassen AF, Cieza A, Sauve K, O'Donnell M, Armstrong R, et al. Comparing contents of outcome measures in cerebral palsy using the International Classification of Functioning (ICF-CY): a systematic review. European Journal of Paediatric Neurology. 2014;18(1):1–12.

[77] Cole AJ, Becker BE. Comprehensive Aquatic Therapy. Butterworth-Heinemann; 2004.

[78] Getz M, Hutzler Y, Vermeer A. The effects of aquatic intervention on perceived physical competence and social acceptance in children with cerebral palsy. European Journal of Special Needs Education. 2007;22(2):217–28.

[79] Lai C-J, Liu W-Y, Yang T-F, Chen C-L, Wu C-Y, Chan R-C. Pediatric aquatic therapy on motor function and enjoyment in children diagnosed with cerebral palsy of various motor severities. Journal of Child Neurology. 2014:0883073814535491.

[80] Jorgić B, Dimitrijević L, Lambeck J, Aleksandrović M, Okičić T, Madić D. Effects of aquatic programs in children and adolescents with cerebral palsy: systematic review. Sport Science. 2012;5(2).

[81] Dimitrijević L, Aleksandrović M, Madić D, Okičić T, Radovanović D, Daly D. The effect of aquatic intervention on the gross motor function and aquatic skills in children with cerebral palsy. Journal of Human Kinetics. 2012;32:167–74.

[82] Getz M, Hutzler Y, Vermeer A, Yarom Y, Unnithan V. The effect of aquatic and land-based training on the metabolic cost of walking and motor performance in children with cerebral palsy: a pilot study. ISRN Rehabilitation. 2012;2012.

[83] Gorter J, Currie S. Aquatic exercise programs for children and adolescents with cerebral palsy: what do we know and where do we go? International Journal of Pediatrics. 2011;2011.

[84] Meregillano G. Hippotherapy. Physical medicine and rehabilitation clinics of north america. 2004;15(4):843–54.

[85] Sterba JA. Does horseback riding therapy or therapist-directed hippotherapy rehabilitate children with cerebral palsy? Developmental Medicine & Child Neurology. 2007;49(1):68–73.

[86] Heine B, Benjamin J. Introduction to hippotherapy. NARHA Strides magazine. 1997;3(2):7.

[87] Tseng S-H, Chen H-C, Tam K-W. Systematic review and meta-analysis of the effect of equine assisted activities and therapies on gross motor outcome in children with cerebral palsy. Disability and Rehabilitation. 2013;35(2):89–99.

[88] Whalen CN, Case-Smith J. Therapeutic effects of horseback riding therapy on gross motor function in children with cerebral palsy: a systematic review. Physical & Occupational Therapy in Pediatrics. 2012;32(3):229–42.

[89] Rosenbaum P, King S, Law M, King G, Evans J. Family-centred service: a conceptual framework and research review. Physical & Occupational Therapy in Pediatrics. 1998;18(1):1–20.

[90] Richards CL, Malouin F. Cerebral palsy: definition, assessment and rehabilitation. Handbook of Clinical Neurology. 2012;111:183–95.

[91] Dirks T, Blauw-Hospers CH, Hulshof LJ, Hadders-Algra M. Differences between the family-centered "COPCA" program and traditional infant physical therapy based on neurodevelopmental treatment principles. Physical Therapy. 2011.

Chapter 5

Strength Training in People with Cerebral Palsy

Cemil Özal, Duygu Türker and Duygu Korkem

Additional information is available at the end of the chapter

http://dx.doi.org/10.5772/64638

Abstract

Disorders affecting muscle strength in children with cerebral palsy (CP) are indicated among the main reasons of the motor performance disorder. Muscle weakness is a common disorder in children with CP and is associated with insufficient or reduced motor unit discharge, inadequate coactivation of antagonist muscles, secondary myopathy, and impaired muscle physiology. Studies have shown the usefulness of strength training in children with CP and revealed the relationship of muscle strength with activity. Strength exercises increase muscle strength, flexibility, posture, and balance in CP. They also increase the level of activity in daily life and develop functional activities.

Keywords: cerebral palsy, muscle strength, strength training, treatment outcome, assessment

1. Introduction

Cerebral palsy (CP) affects activity and social participation in children and is an umbrella term that encompasses permanent and nonprogressive disorders that develop during the prenatal, perinatal, or postnatal period following various effects on the brain that has not yet fully developed [1–7]. This effect on the central nervous system causes disturbances in the neuromuscular, musculoskeletal, and sensory systems of the children, leading to problems related to inadequate posture and motility [8]. These problems then result in decreased independence and physical activity, leading to a sedentary lifestyle and a negative effect on the child's physical development. The spasticity and loss of strength in comparison with their healthy peers in children with CP end in gait disorders and increased energy consumption [9, 10]. The muscle weakness in the trunk and lower extremity is especially important for ambulation and requires strength training [11, 12]. Studies have revealed the positive effects of strength training and the relationship of muscle power with activity in children with CP [5]. Strength training in CP patients leads to increased muscle power, flexibility, posture, and balance. It also increases the activity level during daily living and improves functional activities such as walking and running [6].

We will analyze the factors causing the muscle weakness seen in children with CP in this section. We will also discuss the strength training methods used in the literature, together with the body structure and function in children, activity limitation and participation problems, within the framework of the International Classification of Functioning, Disability and Health: Children & Youth Version (ICF).

2. Definition of pathophysiology of strength inefficiency

Studies have revealed strength loss in the affected extremities of children with CP compared to their peers, even when the child with CP is at a high functional level, and the strength loss increases in correlation with the significance of the neurological effect [13]. The weakness in children with CP can be due to both the disturbed neural mechanisms and the muscle tissue changes. Most investigators believe that the low power production is related to the inadequate coactivation of antagonist muscles, decreased or inadequate motor unit discharge, secondary myopathy and disturbed muscle physiology [5].

2.1. The neurologic basis of weakness

Many neurological factors contribute to the weakness seen in children with CP. Normal neural development is related to progressive strength increase, increased contraction speed, and increased isometric maximum voluntary contraction power. Muscle activity is controlled by the central nervous system via the peripheral nerves. The repetition of normal movement leads to stronger neural networks in the nervous system in healthy children. A normally developing child voluntarily repeats normal activities many times, while a child with CP will repeat abnormal movement patterns, causing strengthening of the abnormal neural networks [14].

The central input that stimulates the motor neurons is decreased in these children due to pyramidal tract damage. The motor neuron pool therefore becomes inadequate in the management of the agonist muscle. The muscle's contraction power is increased both by increasing the number of active motor units and by the firing rate of the already active motor units. This is especially the result of a regular summation pattern of the motor unit, and this arrangement is specific to each muscle. However, motor units work in an inadequate, irregular, and slower than normal manner following upper motor neuron (UMN) damage. The muscle therefore cannot be activated [14, 15].

There is a specific balance between the firing rate and motor unit summation of each muscle during power production. The muscle strength usually develops with the summation of motor units due to the disturbance in the firing rate modulation in spastic muscles. The normal pairing between the motor unit firing rate and the mechanical features of the muscle fibers is also disturbed. This leads to inadequate power production of the muscle and early fatigue [16]. Inadequate firing of motor units leads to strength loss in the early stage, while the decreased motor response adaptation ability limits selective motor control and strength production ability [2]. It has been shown that children with CP are unable to activate the high-threshold motor unit groups necessary for maximum voluntary contraction and are also unable to change the firing rate of the low-threshold motor units [17].

A voluntary movement develops in the agonist muscle, while the antagonist muscle relaxes thanks to the reciprocal inhibitory pathways. The disturbance in the inhibitory pathways leads to abnormal cocontraction. Normal movement requires the prevention of abnormal cocontraction between the agonist and antagonist. The cocontraction seen in children with CP is at a much higher level than in normal children of the same age. These cocontractions especially develop during rapid reciprocal movements [18, 19].

The sensory and motor innervation of the muscle spindle is complicated. The muscle spindle structure is very sensitive to the length of the muscle. The stimulation threshold of the sensory fibers of the muscle spindle can lead to a response of zero in the chronically shortened spastic muscle, while, in contrast, it can cause abnormal relaxation length and decreased control of upper centers via the afferent fibers of the muscle spindle in the chronically elongated muscle. There is marked agonist weakness in children with CP due to prolonged spastic antagonist muscle activity [14].

In short, the neural factors that cause muscle weakness in children with CP are decreased motor management, stronger abnormal neural networks, disturbed firing pattern, reciprocal inhibition, and disturbance in the adjustment within the muscle spindle. The neurophysiological abnormalities in children with CP cause persistent and permanent problems when passing into adulthood. These abnormalities limit the ability of children with CP to grow so that he/she can become stronger in the normal manner [14].

2.2. The muscular basis of weakness

In the past, it was believed that muscle tissue histology would not change in a subject with a brain lesion. Recent studies have revealed that the disturbances in the morphological structure of the skeletal muscle in children with CP cause muscular weakness [14]. Sinkjaer et al. [20] have demonstrated that the muscle tissue can show histopathological changes after an UMN lesion. The muscle tissue changes vary according to the child's age and ambulatory level. The age of cerebral damage can also affect the histology [21].

2.2.1. The changes seen in the muscle fiber types

It has been reported that motor unit types can change following an UMN lesion. The activity and size of the motor neuron largely determines the number of muscle fibers in a motor unit and the type of myosin within these fibers. Myosin production is modulated with hormonal and mechanical activity. There are various ratios of type I and type II motor units in most muscles used in movement, and these ratios vary according to the basic function of the muscle. For example, M. Soleus mostly contains slow contracting type I fibers and supports posture

M. Gastrocnemius mostly has fast contracting type II fibers and therefore provides the pushing power for walking and running. The neural input that is disturbed because of cerebral damage affects the differentiation of these fiber types. With growth, adult myosin forms take the place of the embryonic and neonatal forms, changing the muscle. This change takes place from childhood to adulthood. The muscle is modeled according to the activity level, environmental effects, and especially mechanical tension. The disturbed activity level and ability to transfer load affect myosin development [14, 21].

Muscle spindle development and synthesis of acetylcholine receptors depend on the neural activation pattern in the prenatal period. Neural lesions developing in the prenatal period can disturb the development of fetal muscle cells, muscle spindles, and neurotransmission. The child can therefore be born with inadequately differentiated muscle tissue and possible structural abnormalities in the muscle spindle and acetylcholine receptors. The first weeks of the postnatal period where there are marked changes in the neuromuscular and terminal connections are critical for muscle physiology and development. Delayed maturation in postnatal muscle fiber development has been shown in 21 low birthweight children with an UMN lesion. The changes in the muscle contractile features in children with CP are characterized by predominant type I and selective type II (a) and (b) atrophy. An increase in the number of type I fibers in these children leads to low power in the elongated muscle without the ability to produce contractions that rapidly produce a high degree of power [14].

2.2.2. Changes in muscle fiber length

Maximum power depends on the optimum interaction of actin and myosin filaments, and muscle power is related to the number of sarcomeres and the length of each sarcomere [22]. Fiber growth is a response to bone growth and loading. The tension in children with CP that develops due to the elongated sarcomeres decreases the interaction between the actin and myosin filaments, limiting the number of cross-bridges that develop and the force production ability [14].

Studies on children with CP have found sarcomere lengths to be abnormally long compared to a control group without spasticity. It has been reported that only 40% of the normal power can be produced with elongated sarcomeres [14, 23].

2.2.3. Changes in the total muscle length

The fascicle length is shorter in children with CP than in healthy peers. This may be due to the disturbance in volume, fibril atrophy, decreased pennation angle, and shortening of the intramuscular aponeurosis. Malaiya et al. [24] have compared the medial M. Gastrocnemius in 16 preadolescent spastic hemiparetic and 15 healthy children. They have only found that the hemiparetic side muscle fascicle length was 10% shorter than in healthy children during the ankle resting phase. Besides the most bulging part of the muscle being shorter, the musculotendinous unit tendon was longer than normal. Shorter muscles contain less sarcomeres and therefore have less cross-bridges to produce power. A longer tendon decreases the biomechanical benefit [14].

http://dx.doi.org/10.5772/64638

Although the spastic muscle tries to produce maximum power over the length-tension curve, the functional capacity is decreased. The reason is that the spastic muscle cannot work for prolonged periods at the optimum length needed to produce muscle function [14]. Increased power production during the push-off phase has been shown following M. Gastrocnemius fascia lengthening surgery in children with CP. This is because the lengthened spastic muscle works mostly from the middle point instead of the endpoint or the longer muscle is less sensitive to the reflex response at the early stage of the movement. The person can therefore produce voluntary contraction during the push-off phase [25].

The spastic muscle is short, and the antagonist muscle is therefore chronically in the rest position. A muscle in the rest position has a biomechanical disadvantage as it cannot shorten adequately to produce the necessary functional movement and create effective power [14].

2.2.4. *Changes in muscle cross-sectional area*

The capacity of the muscle to produce power is directly related to its cross-sectional area. Every unit of the cross-sectional area takes its expected adult form with growth, approximately after puberty. Strength training results can therefore be affected by the child's age [14]. Marbini et al. [26] have shown that children with CP have a decrease in the M. Triceps surae and adductor muscle cross-sectional area and pennation angle. The volume of the M. Gastrocnemius medialis with a decreased pennation angle is 30% less than normal [14]. The muscle fiber may never develop in premature children compared to a term child, and the cross-sectional area is therefore lower than normal and maximum contraction is limited. Studies have shown that muscle volume is lower in children with CP; cross-sectional area and intramuscular adipose tissue are increased compared to normal peers [14].

2.2.5. *Changes in the passive features of the muscles*

The amount of collagen is increased in the muscles of children with CP. The collagen amount is increased in relation to an increased degree of disturbance. This is responsible for contracture development. The muscle's passive viscoelastic features are affected by the collagen type, amount, collagen connections, and structural organization of the collagen fibers. This influences the internal resistance during viscoelastic contraction and the passive resistance during elongation in contraction in the opposite direction that the muscle has to put up with. A weak agonist muscle may not allow full lengthening of the spastic antagonist and may lead to contracture development. Increased passive tension therefore leads to muscle weakness [14].

In short, the muscular factors that cause the muscle weakness in children with CP are the disturbance in myosin production, structural abnormalities in the perinatal period, decreased muscle fascicle length, increased sarcomere length, decreased muscle volume, and decreased physiological section area [14].

3. The assessment of muscle strength in people with cerebral palsy

The assessment of muscle strength in children with CP has become standard in clinical application and research. The muscle power has a different distribution in many children and adolescents with CP, and this can lead to difficulties in the realization of daily functional activities [27]. Recent studies have shown that children with CP can benefit from strength training programs [12, 28–31]. Clinicians and investigators interested in the effect of strength training programs should therefore have adequate knowledge on the psychometric features of strength measurements in these children [27].

There are three different muscle strength measurements used in children and adolescents with CP in general: isometric, isokinetic, and functional strength test. The isometric-based test measures the power production ability of a muscle group without causing a change in the general muscle-tendon length. A maximal isometric contraction is only an indicator of the power production capacity in that particular condition and with the current muscle length and does not cause any difference in the muscle length during the task. Other factors accompanying muscle weakness such as excessive cocontraction and selective motor control disturbance can inhibit the ability to produce agonist power. However, the measured strength in many children with CP can significantly increase not only with repeated exercise but also with strength training. This is a major factor in evaluating weakness in CP and makes the validity of testing strength in CP or other spastic disorders doubtful. Isokinetic, the other measurement type, means 'same speed' and indicates tests performed at a predefined constant speed [27].

There are some administrative difficulties related to measuring strength in children with CP. The person being evaluated should be able to understand what he/she needs to do to produce maximum effort and conform with this repeatedly. The test positions require some modification in these individuals due to the short muscles, and the examining person needs to be careful not to applying counter force at the joint contracture point. Test positions that promote or inhibit the use of flexion or extension synergies can also have various effects on the power values from CP patients. Poor selective control in some muscle groups can prevent an individual from performing a task. Motor control limitations are probably not an important factor in the ability to generate power in CP children, as they are of lower intensity. As an example, when evaluating the lower extremity power in children with mild or moderate spastic diplegia or hemiplegia that have been tested in many muscle groups, what was understood from the task of selective control was the test position and the ankle dorsiflexors as a single muscle group and these were tested only in 2 of the 30 participants during knee extension [11]. However, motor control disorders can hinder a comprehensive strength test and training in those with more prominent neurological involvement [27].

3.1. Manual muscle testing—portable manual dynamometry

Muscle strength is usually evaluated with methods bases on isometric resistance in clinical practice [32]. Two methods used to evaluate muscle power are the manual muscle test (MMT) and manual dynamometry. MMT uses the 6-point (0–5) Medical Research Council (MRC) scale. However, the ability to determine muscle power changes with MMT is especially poor

http://dx.doi.org/10.5772/64638

in grades 4 and 5 [33, 34]. MMT is a simple manual instrument that has a small internal load cell that can measure muscle strength (in Newton) [27]. Portable manual dynamometry (PMD) has been shown to be a reliable and easy-to-use method to measure muscle strength in clinical practice. PMD enables the measurement of isometric contraction [35]. Two types of measurement methods have been defined [32]. In the make test, the examiner keeps the dynamometer in a fixed position, while the subject pushes against the dynamometer. In the break test, the examiner pushes the dynamometer against the subject's limb until the maximal effort of the subject is overcome and the joint cannot resist [35]. The make test has been shown to be more reliable than the break test. Testing arm muscles is more reliable than testing leg muscles and the affected side values are higher than the unaffected side in hemiparesis patients. It is very important for the examiner to have adequate muscle strength to hold the PMD stable [32].

3.2. Isokinetic dynamometry

Isokinetic dynamometry is usually performed in a laboratory setting, and a computer-controlled device is used to measure the muscle power created during a controlled movement. Isometric resistance is used to determine the strength of a muscle group around a joint with limited range of motion (ROM) but does not provide detailed information on the dynamic qualities of muscle strength during full ROM. This information can be obtained with dynamic instruments such as isokinetic machines. Isokinetic devices enable full and reliable monitorization of individual muscle development during a training program even when the muscle power is very limited. Isokinetic muscle training had a certain advantage to other types of strength training as the largest rotational moment is created throughout the full ROM. Isokinetic dynamometers are also relatively more reliable as resistance is adjusted according to participant effort with a measurement device. The resistance is therefore decreased immediately and the risk of injury minimized when limiting factors such as pain or discomfort are suddenly experienced. The isokinetic instrument shows the strength curves throughout ROM and provides visual feedback to the administrator. This feature is valuable in the motor development of children with minor disability and also in those with normal intelligence. There is only limited information on the reliability of isokinetic tests in subjects with neurological disorders. The reliability of isokinetic strength measurements at higher angular speeds has also not been determined. High angular speeds are typical of daily and sports activities and should therefore be included for follow-up and motivation purposes in the exercise protocols of children with CP who frequently display proprioceptive or attentive disorders. The main point in selecting a measurement method is reliability [36]. The reliability in testing the isokinetic power of knee flexors and extensors has mostly been shown for adult participants without CP in the literature. It has been reported that the test procedures are highly reliable at a great many angular speeds for the concentric contraction of knee extensors and flexors [37]. Molnar et al. [38] have discussed the reliability of the isokinetic tests of many muscle groups in the upper and lower extremities in children aged 7–15 years. They concluded that performing isokinetic tests was simple and highly reliable in children with a low-grade learning disability, as much as those with normal intelligence, who were typically developing children.

3.3. Functional strength testing

Functional strength tests: It is important to use functional exercises to test functional performance in the large muscle groups that are essential for standing and walking in children with CP. The following are three closed kinetic chain exercises [27, 39]:

The Lateral Step Test (on a 20-cm bench): This test is used to evaluate lower extremity muscle performance. The subject is asked to stand on the tested extremity with the feet parallel and the shoulders separated. The proper lateral step technique is defined as achieving a position within knee extension for the tested extremity during the test's extension phase. The number of times the untested foot's heel or toes touch the ground is counted. The test-retest reliability has been found to be excellent in young and healthy adult subjects. This protocol has not been previously evaluated in patients with CP [27, 40].

Sit-stand up (from 90°knee and hip flexion to the standing position): This is a functional test and the child must be able to stand up without using his hands. The child is put on a small bench and sits down with the feet on the ground and the knees flexed 90°. The child has to be able to stand up without using the hands and without any help from the bench with the arms or body during the transition. The repetitions where the child's legs and hips are within 15° of the extension position are counted [27, 39].

Attain stand thought half knell without using the arms: This is a functional test and the child must be able to stand up without using his arms. The child is put on a pillow in the high kneeling position, leaving the hands free. This means the weight is supported by one knee and the foot of the other side and that the alignment can change as long as the hips are away from the area below the legs and/or the weight-bearing surface. The child is told to stand up without any external support from a piece of furniture or the floor. The repetitions are counted every time the child succeeds in attaining the standing position, and both legs and hips were within 15° of the extension position [27, 39].

4. Strength training in people with cerebral palsy

Strength training was not at the forefront for children with CP until recently because it was believed it would increase spasticity. However, this has not been supported by the previously uncontrolled studies showing that strength training can increase lower extremity muscle power without increasing spasticity in these children [41, 42]. Several studies have provided adequate evidence for its effect on muscle power, but these effects have probably been overestimated due to the lower methodological quality of these studies [30, 43]. A few uncontrolled studies on the effect of strength training on motility results in children with CP have reported a limited effect [28, 41]. Three randomized clinical reviews published recently have evaluated both muscle power and motility in CP children, but conflicting results have been reported [44–46]. One of the explanations for these conflicting results could be the significant differences in training characteristics such as the type, intensity, and duration. The training should be customized for it to be successful and should stimulate more than the increase obtained with intensity as it does not include it [47].

http://dx.doi.org/10.5772/64638

4.1. Isokinetic training

Isokinetic resistance training has been made possible with mechanical devices such as Cybex II that keep extremity movement at a predefined constant speed. The resistance from the isokinetic device is produced in proportion to the applied force. Increased speed is therefore met by increased resistance. The maximum voluntary effort is met by the maximum resistance within the range of motion. More markedly, isokinetic resistance exercises have been found to be an excellent and safe training type to increase both the strength and power in reciprocal movement templates [48]. The measurements made with the Cybex II, the device used in this study, have also been found to be very reliable. Resistance training is used by athletes with cerebral palsy. The athletes are trained to compete in lifting weights at the cerebral palsy games, an approved activity. However, advocates of the specified treatment approach feel that weight training could be detrimental for persons with cerebral palsy. The potential harmful effects include increased resting muscle tonus, increased abnormal standing position, and decreased range of motion. Studies have shown that subjects with cerebral palsy experience increased strength with systematic resistance exercises. However, there is no study on the effect of systematic resistance exercises on movement function in these subjects. Increased motor function can also be gained through repetitive attempts without any resistance. Training results in more effective muscle activity as shown in electromyography records following a series of training attempts. All the repeated training attempts have been performed with normal subjects, and there are no studies on subjects with cerebral palsy. The merging of developments seen in nerve-muscle performance after repeated exercises without any resistance in unrelated persons with the known nerve-muscle problems in CP indicates a need for experimental research in this area [30, 45, 47–49].

It is recommended that for children with cerebral palsy, the following methods of strengthening be considered
Isokinetic training
Progressive resistance exercise
Bicycle and treadmill exercises
Weight training
Upper extremity strengthening
Aquatic training
Sports and recreation
Electrotherapy

4.2. Progressive resistance exercise

Progressive resistance exercise (PRE) training is a well-established strength training method where intensity is gradually increased. This stimulates more strength gain than related to typical growth and development [50].

The main elements of PRE are as follows: Providing enough resistance so that a low number of repetitions [usually 8–12] can be completed before fatigue starts, increasing the amount of resistance progressively as the strength increases and continuing the training program for an adequate duration so that its benefits are seen [50].

There have been recommendations to avoid strength training in children with CP in the past because it would increase spasticity, decrease ROM, and increase problems with walking. Systematic reviews have provided increasing evidence that strength training in children with CP increases muscle power without any side effects related to spasticity or ROM [30, 51, 52]. However, a recent review's authors concluded that strength training is not effective in children with CP [5]. It has also not been possible to make a decision on whether strength training is effective in improving functions such as the ability to walk. As expected, muscle strength decreases 6 weeks after the conclusion of the training and this has also been observed in healthy children [53]. Surprisingly, this effect has not been observed in a few comparable studies (mostly uncontrolled) with follow-up evaluations in children with CP [14, 41, 45]. Based on the results of controlled studies, it can be recommended to include strengthening in a regular exercise routine to enable increased strength levels [54].

Daily activities only need a specific amount of muscle power (i.e., the lowest threshold). There may be increases in these lowest threshold levels and movements, but there may also be increased strength that does not provide an additional advantage for movement improvement (i.e., the highest threshold) [55]. Strength training will therefore not be the appropriate treatment option if the aim is to improve mobility. Other components such as balance and coordination may affect the improvement in motility more than muscle power by itself [56].

The 12-week functional PRE strength training has been shown to be effective in increasing the strength of the knee extensors and hip abductor by 11–12% and the six-repetition maximum leg strength by 14%. However, this strength increase does not result in increased motility. In conclusion, functional PRE is said to be effective in increasing leg muscle strength in children with CP. PRE can also be included in a more intensive treatment regime or can be used as a target treatment after waiting for temporary muscle weakness as seen before or after botulinum toxin A or surgical treatment [56]. A typical PRE program for individuals with CP consisted of 2–4 exercises where isokinetic dynamometers, weight machines, or free weights were used. The participants typically completed three or four sets with 5–10 repeats of each exercise with 50–65% training intensity of one-repetition maximum. They were usually trained for three times a week for a duration ranging from 6 to 10 weeks. Studies vary greatly on the types of participants and have included children and adults aged 4–47 years with spastic hemiplegia, diplegia or quadriplegia alone or in combination and also a few patients with ataxia or dystonia [57].

4.3. Bicycle and treadmill exercises

Children with CP suffer from weakness and low endurance [11, 18]. The size of the effect for strength changes has varied greatly between studies. This variability in results could be due to the method-related differences in intervention intensity, frequency, and duration [58]. Bicycle riding is a rehabilitation tool commonly used in physiotherapy to improve power and cardiovascular form and is recommended to individuals with CP as an appropriate exercise to keep in shape [59]. Stationary bicycle programs can provide resistance exercises for lower extremity muscles [58]. More studies are needed on stationary bicycle interventions for children with CP, but they have the potential to improve strength and cardiovascular form with minimum conditions for balance and motor control.

Treadmill training with partial body weight support (TTPBWS) is becoming more popular in the rehabilitation of children with CP. The literature on TTPBWS in CP mainly consists of case reports and small nonrandomized studies without a control group. Three separate reviews of TTPBWS in children with CP and also one on TTPBWS in pediatric rehabilitation have been published recently. Two reviews have concluded that TTPBWS can be safe and effective in increasing walking speed, while one review has stated that it could be useful to improve gross motor skills [60]. On the other hand, another review has concluded that there is not enough evidence to determine whether TTPBWS leads to an improvement in children with CP, that the evidence is for results in children with CP is weak, and that randomized studies are required to evaluate issues such as efficacy and dose [61]. These reviews have recommended more definite studies to determine the effectiveness of TTPBWS for children with CP. TTPBWS has also been reported to lead to changes in gait spatiotemporal parameters [62, 63].

The use of a mechanical treadmill can improve walking in children with CP skills [60]. Walking on a treadmill provides an opportunity for repeated training in the total gait cycle, facilitates the advanced gait model, and decreases the effect of poor balance on the child's ability to lift weights during walking when a body weight-supporting system is used [60, 61, 64].

Some preliminary studies have reported that TTPBWS is possible in children with CP as young as 15 months and that it can even be used in children who cannot yet walk independently [65]. Developing the gait has the potential to increase mobility and have a positive effect on the home, school, and wider community social participation of children with CP.

Treadmill training seems to be effective in the improvement of general gross motor skills. Different studies have evaluated the effects of treadmill training on gross motor skills. They have all reported important changes in the gross motor function measurement (GMFM) dimension (walking, running, jumping) after finding a major effect in the two groups skills [60].

According to a study has evaluated the effect of treadmill training on the energy consumption (EC), which evaluates the energy cost of walking. A large effect size for change was found in the EC when the progress in all participants was recorded [62].

4.4. Weight training

Although strength training seems to be safe for children of all ages when performed appropriately, loads should not be over the maximum before physical growth is completed for protect harmful effects on musculoskeletal tissues. Other safety issues include a more progressive accumulation of resistance, especially in weak children, that does not permit lifting weights by a child without supervision or hanging a weight from an extremity without muscular effort or external support. The child should not train on the same muscle groups on consecutive days. The protocol needs to be changed if there is excessive or continuing pain due to the strengthening program or if muscle stiffness increased [66].

4.5. Upper extremity strengthening

Upper extremity muscle weakness is clinically important in children with CP as it is related to function. There is also evidence that upper extremity muscle weakness decreases the ability to perform daily living activities in children with CP [14, 67–69].

Muscle strengthening in individuals with CP is a general treatment intervention to increase strength and function, and it can be presented as a separate training or combined with other intervention types such as electrical stimulation, botulinum toxin A (BoNTA), aerobic training, or motor training [47, 70, 71]. Scianni et al. [5] and Franki et al. [72] have reported that muscle strengthening in CP will not increase muscle spasticity in their review. This has also been demonstrated in studies on upper extremity strengthening. Individuals with CP need consistent upper extremity training because CP can lead to muscle contractures and functional disturbance [73]. Considering that the poor muscle strength in children with CP in one of the most important factors affecting motor function, increasing muscle strength is a fundamental treatment for motor performance [30]. However, the number of studies on improving upper extremity functions through active physical training of the upper extremities in CP is limited [74]. These studies have recommended strength training with intensive repetitions that develop upper extremity exercise capacity as rehabilitation treatment in children with CP.

4.6. Aquatic training

The special characteristics of water provide a desired environment for children and adolescents with CP [75, 76]. For example, the weight lifting conditions are better in water with decreased body control amount, joint load, and effect of gravity. In conclusion, the aquatic physical activity protects joint integrity more than conditions outside [77]. Studies have shown that performing motor skills in the water will probably increase confidence and needs less resistance to try difficult tasks when compared with training on land [77]. Activities in water can also be more fun and different for children, possibly increasing motivation and interest. Aquatic physical activity can be significantly beneficial for persons with higher gross motor function classification system (GMFCS) levels and marked movement limitations who may have more difficulty and be more restricted in performing physical activities outside water [75]. It must be noted that there are only a limited number of programs outside water for this population [78].

The presence of aquatic facilities and the high degree of acceptance by the general public have led to significant interest by children and adolescents with CP in aquatic programs [79]. In 2010, Brunton and Bartlett described the participation of adolescents with CP in exercise programs. They reported swimming as one of the activities most liked by the participants; it was the second and third most common activity for GMFCS levels I, II and III and more significantly, the most common activity for the higher GMFCS levels of IV and V [80]. Similarly, Zwier et al. [81] reported that swimming was the second most common activity for children with CP aged five to seven years and that 71% of these children were involved in swimming. In short, aquatic activities can be lifelong beneficial exercises and physical activities in these subjects. There is also evidence that this population with physical and cognitive skills already participates in aquatic activities [75].

However, aquatic activity programs for this population are few in number and the effects of these interventions have not therefore been effectively evaluated in subjects with CP. Kelly and Darrah have reported in 2005 that aquatic exercise has many observed benefits on flexibility, respiratory function, muscle power, and gross motor function, but there are very few studies on its effects. The authors have included three articles in their review, but the information is limited by the poor methodological quality. They concluded that 'More evidence is needed on the effect of aquatic exercises on keeping children with CP in shape and on their place in physical management programs' [75].

4.7. Sports and recreation

Childhood and adolescence are important period when disabled youngsters develop self-confidence and their attitudes and behaviors to transfer to adulthood [82]. Play, recreation, and sports participation have important effects on general development and are essential elements for childhood and adolescence [83, 84].

Sports and recreation have many physiological benefits thanks to regular participation in physical activities during childhood and adolescence, in addition to their psychosocial benefits. These include the increased muscle density and fat-free muscle tissue in adulthood, better management of body weight, low risk for high blood pressure and decreased feelings of depression and social isolation [85].

Despite physiological and psychosocial benefits, the rate of physical inactivity among disabled children is much higher than those without a disability and many specialists believe that this can eventually lead to health problems in adulthood [86–88].

4.8. Electrotherapy

Those who advocate electrotherapy applications state that electrical stimulation (ES) increases strength and motor function and is an attractive alternative for strengthening children with CP with poor selective motor control [89]. Although there are instances where ES can be used for its positive effect, it is usually included in rehabilitation approaches as a complementary element [90].

ES can be used in children with CP and adolescents to increase muscle power, improve functional capacity, and to teach the muscle its new function and strengthen it following orthopedic interventions. Neuromuscular electrical stimulation (NMES) and threshold electrical stimulation (TES) are commonly used variations [89]. NMES is application of an electrical stimulus to the lower motor neuron or terminal branches to cause depolarization and finally muscle contraction [91]. The strength increase in NMES develops with two mechanisms. The first one is the loading principle; the muscle's strength is increased with increased cross-sectional area of the muscle. In the second mechanism, selective development of type II fibers enables synaptic activity development in the muscle [92].

The use of neuromuscular stimulation for a functional target is also known as functional electrical stimulation (FES) [92]. FES can be defined as the electrical stimulation of the nerve or muscle to produce the desired joint movement when a motor task is being realized and can also be used to improve the underlying motor control by increasing the specific task motion repetition [93, 94].

NMES-type currents administered to the agonist muscle have been proven to both strengthen the motor unit and increase contractile proteins, resulting in muscle hypertrophy and thus contributing to a stronger muscle [92]. FES can affect the potential of interneurons and motor neurons to be stimulated and provide sensory input at the same time and therefore contribute to individuals producing more power than they could voluntarily [95, 96]. Children with CP have been demonstrated to show beneficial development in muscle power and muscle cross-sectional area following NMES administration [97, 98].

Alternatively, TES is the administration of a low-intensity (2–10 mA) and long-duration (8–12 h) electrical current to the muscles during sleep. It does not cause visible muscle contractions. It basically increases local blood flow and enables vascularization of atrophic muscles, increasing muscle mass, and endurance [99]. Results evaluating the effect of TES on muscle power and function have emphasized that there is no gain in function or muscle power or muscle cross section in children who underwent TES treatment [100–102].

ES parameters used in children with CP reveals the following: frequencies were generally in the range 30 to 45 Hz, pulse durations 100–300 μs, and the time taken to reach the desired intensity (ramp up) ranged from 0.5 to 2 sec. Some variation existed in the contraction/relaxation times for the activation of the muscles. The TES on: off times were generally equal; however, with NMES, some authors used equal times and others ensured that the 'off' time was at least double the 'on' time. The intensity of stimulation and duration of treatment depended on whether TES or NMES was employed, with TES tending to be applied for a minimum of 30 h per week for 6–17 months. NMES was most commonly applied for 15–20 min per week in a task-orientated therapy setting or for up to 1 h daily for 2 months when applied at home [89].

5. Strength training within the framework of ICF

The positive and negative results of strength training have been evaluated with the use of the International Classification of Functioning, Disability and Health that provides a framework for the definition of health [30]. It is possible to define the disorder in the person according to impairment, activity restriction, and participation limitations in this scope. According to the ICF definition, impairment is deviation or losses of body function or structure, activity restrictions are difficulties in performing tasks or actions, and participation limitations are problems related to life conditions. A person's functionality and disability is thought to be a dynamic interaction between contextual factors such as the environment and the person's health condition [30].

5.1. Impairment

There is no evidence that strength training increases spasticity and contractures in individuals with CP. Some clinicians have postulated that spastic CP individuals are not weak and that the disturbed performance of functional activities that is observed is actually a result of the spasticity [103]. Depending on clinical observations, it has been said that the increased effort related to strength training can increase spasticity in patients with a neurological disorder and that this can lead to increased muscle and joint contractures and decreased motor function [30]. However, this opinion has not been supported by the literature. Studies on the effect on strength training on spasticity have either found no effect or have even shown it could potentially decrease spasticity. Similarly, there is no evidence that strengthening programs will decrease ROM in individuals with CP; evidence even suggests that strength training can increase ROM, especially in the lower extremities [30].

5.2. Activity

A strengthening program planned to increase muscle strength could be expected to have less effect on the measurement of muscle power than on activity measurements as other factors such as sensory function, coordination, and even psychological factors contribute to motor performance [30]. Significant increases in the D and E dimensions of the GMFM have been found following a strengthening program aimed at lower extremity muscles [31]. These parts of the GMFM activities measure for example standing on one leg, standing up from a sitting position, walking, running, kicking, jumping, and walking up and down the steps [28] In relation to gait speed, a study has found a positive effect after strengthening, while another has found no change. This indicates that strengthening programs that have been developed into a form suitable for individual requirements can provide better functional results than less customized programs [31, 104]. Upper extremity strengthening exercises can also increase the endurance of children with CP using a wheelchair [30].

5.3. Participation

There are only a few studies evaluating the effect of strength training on the social participation of individuals with CP. However, it has anecdotally been reported that some participants have felt confident enough to join a regular community exercise program after the training was completed [105, 106].

5.4. Contextual factors

Contextual factors are an important point in evaluating the effects of strengthening programs. Clinicians need information on the effects of various environmental and personal contextual factors so that they can administer the best program. Despite the importance of these contextual factors, the information in the included articles is inadequate to obtain a meaningful result [30].

6. Conclusion

Since muscle weakness is a common disorder in children with CP, muscle strength may influence motor performance which affects activity in daily life and develop functional activities. Muscle weakness might resulted by the neurologic or the muscular basis. Muscle strength can measure with several clinical tests included isometric, isokinetic, and functional strength test. Strength interventions include different ways such as isokinetic training, progressive resistance exercise, bicycle and treadmill exercises, weight training, upper extremity strengthening, aquatic training, sports and recreation and electrotherapy. Strength training in CP has beneficial effects on body structure and function, activity limitation, and participation problems according to ICF in children with CP. In the literature, more studies needed for improved evidence-based clinical interventions.

Author details

Cemil Özal*, Duygu Türker and Duygu Korkem

*Address all correspondence to: cemilozal@hotmail.com

Department of Physiotherapy and Rehabilitation, Institute of Health Sciences, Hacettepe University, Ankara, Turkey

References

[1] Giuliani CA. Dorsal rhizotomy for children with cerebral palsy: support for concepts of motor control. Phys Ther. 1991;71:248–59.

[2] Damiano DL, Quinlivan J, Owen BF, Shaffrey M, Abel MF. Spasticity versus strength in cerebral palsy: relationships among involuntary resistance, voluntary torque and motor function. Eur J Neurol Off Eur Federat Neurol Soc. 2001;8(5):40–9.

[3] Engsberg JR, Ross SA, Olree KS, Park TS. Ankle spasticity and strength in children with spastic diplegic cerebral palsy. Dev Med Child Neurol. 2000;42(1):42–7.

[4] Engsberg JR, Ross SA. Hip spasticity and strength in children with spastic diplegia cerebral palsy. J Appl Biomech. 2000;16:221–33.

[5] Scianni A, Butler JM, Ada L, Teixeira-Salmela LF. Muscle strengthening is not effective in children and adolescents with cerebral palsy: a systematic review. Aust J Physiother. 2009;55:81–7.

[6] McBurney H, Taylor NF, Dodd KJ, Graham HK. A qualitative analysis of the benefits of strength training for young people with cerebral palsy. Dev Med Child Neurol. 2003;45(10):658–63.

[7] Bax M, Goldstein M, Rosenbaum P, Leviton A, Paneth N, Dan B, et al. Proposed definition and classification of cerebral palsy, April 2005. Dev Med Child Neurol. 2005;47(8):571–6.

[8] Livanelioğlu A, Günel, MK. Serebral Palside Fizyoterapi. Ankara: Yeni Özbek Matbaası.; 2009.

[9] Orlin MN, Palisano RJ, Chiarello LA, et al. Participation in home, extracurricular, and community activities among children and young people with cerebral palsy. Dev Med Child Neurol. 2010;52(2):160–6.

[10] Koman AL, Smith BP, Shilt JS. Cerebral palsy. Lancet. 2004;363:1619–28.

[11] Wiley ME, Damiano DL. Lower-extremity strength profiles in spastic cerebral palsy. Dev Med Child Neurol. 1998;40(2):100–7.

[12] Damiano DL, Vaughan CL, Abel MF. Muscle response to heavy resistance exercise in children with spastic cerebral palsy. Dev Med Child Neurol. 1995;37:731–9.

[13] Finlay H, Ainscough J, Craig J. Current clinical practice in the use of muscle strengthening in children and young people with cerebral palsy – a regional survey of Paediatric Physiotherapists. APCP J. 2012;3(1):27–41.

[14] Mockford M, Caulton JM. The pathophysiological basis of weakness in children with cerebral palsy. Pediatr Phys Ther. 2010;22(2):222–33.

[15] Stackhouse SK, Binder-Macleod SA, Lee SC. Voluntary muscle activation, contractile properties and fatigability in children with and without cerebral palsy. Muscle Nerve. 2005;31(5):594–601.

[16] Rose J, McGill KC. The motor unit in cerebral palsy. Dev Med Child Neurol. 1998;40(4): 270–7.

[17] Rose J, McGill KC. Neuromuscular activation and motor-unit firing characteristics in cerebral palsy. Dev Med Child Neurol. 2005;47(5):329–36.

[18] Elder GC, Kirk J, Stewart G, Cook K, Weir D, Marshall A, Leahey L. Contributing factors to muscle weakness in children with cerebral palsy. Dev Med Child Neurol. 2003;45(8): 542–50.

[19] Givon U. Muscle weakness in cerebral palsy. Acta Orthop Traumatol Turc. 2009;43(2): 87–93.

[20] Sinkjaer T, Magnussen I. Passive, intrinsic and reflex-mediated stiffness in the ankle extensors of hemiparetic patients. Brain. 1994;117(Pt 2):355–63.

[21] Ito J, Araki A, Tanaka H, Tasaki T, Cho K, Yamazaki R. Muscle histopathology in spastic cerebral palsy. Brain Dev. 1996;18(4):299–303.

[22] Lieber RL, Steinman S, Barash IA, Chambers H. Structural and functional changes in spastic skeletal muscle. Muscle Nerve. 2004;29(5):615–27.

[23] Lieber RL, Friden J. Spasticity causes a fundamental rearrangement of muscle-joint interaction. Muscle Nerve. 2002;24:256–70.

[24] Malaiya R, McNee AE, Fry NR, Eve LC, Gough M, Shortland AP. The morphology of the medial gastrocnemius in typically developing children and children with spastic hemiplegic cerebral palsy. J Electromyogr Kinesiol. 2007;17(6):657–63.

[25] Rose SA, DeLuca PA, Davis III RB, Ounpuu S, Gage JR. Kinematic and kinetic evaluation of the ankle after lengthening of the gastrocnemius fascia in children with cerebral palsy. J Pediatr Orthop. 1993;13(6):727–32.

[26] Marbini A, Ferrari A, Cioni G, Bellanova MF, Fusco C, Gemignani F. Immunohistochemical study of muscle biopsy in children with cerebral palsy. Brain Dev. 2002;24(2): 63–6.

[27] Verschuren O, Ketelaar M, Takken T, Van Brussel M, Helders PMJ, Gorter JM. Reliability of hand-held dynamometry and functional strength tests for the lower extremity in children with cerebral palsy. Disabil Rehabil. 2008;30(18):1358–66.

[28] Damiano DL, Abel MF. Functional outcomes of strength training in spastic cerebral palsy. Arch Phys Med Rehabil. 1998;79:119–25.

[29] Darrah J, Wessel J, Nearinburg P, O'Connor M. Evaluation of a community fitness program for adolescents with cerebral palsy. Ped Phys Ther. 1999;11:18–23.

[30] Dodd KJ, Taylor NF, Damiano DL. A systematic review of the effectiveness of strength-training programs for people with cerebral palsy. Arch Phys Med Rehabil. 2002;83:1157–64.

[31] MacPhail HE, Kramer JF. Effect of isokinetic strength-training on functional ability and walking efficiency in adolescents with cerebral palsy. Dev Med Child Neurol. 1995;37(9):763–75.

[32] Eek MN, Kroksmark AK, Beckung E. Isometric muscle torque in children 5 to 15 years of age: normative data. Arch Phys Med Rehabil. 2006;87:1091–9.

[33] Schwartz S, Cohen ME, Herbison GJ, Shah A. Relationship between two measures of upper extremity strength: manual muscle test compared to hand-held myometry. Arch Phys Med Rehabil. 1992;73:1063–68.

[34] Aitkens S, Lord J, Bernauer E, Fowler WM, Lieberman JS, Berck P. Relationship of manual muscle testing to objective strength measurements. Muscle Nerve. 1989;12:173.

[35] Stratford PW, Balsor BE. A comparison of make and break tests using a hand-held dynamometer and the Kin-Com. J Orthop Sports Phys Ther. 1994;19:28–32.

[36] Ayalon M, Ben-Sira D, Hutzler Y, Gilad T. Reliability of isokinetic strength measurements of the knee in children with cerebral palsy. Dev Med Child Neurol. 2000;42:398–402.

[37] Perrin DH. Isokinetic Exercise and Assessment. Champain, IL: Human Kinetics Publishers; 1993.

[38] Molnar GE, Alexander J, Gutfeld N. Reliability of quantitative strength measurements in children. Arch Phys Med Rehabil 1979;60:218–221

[39] Gage JR. Gait analysis: an essential tool in the treatment of cerebral palsy. Clin Orthoped. 1993;288:126–34.

[40] Worrell TW, Borchert B, Erner K, Fritz J, Leerar P. Effect of a lateral step-up exercise protocol on quadriceps and lower extremity performance. J Orthop Sports Phys Ther. 1993;18(6):646–53.

[41] Morton JF, Brownlee M, McFadyen AK. The effects of progressive resistance training for children with cerebral palsy. Clin Rehabil. 2005;19:283–9.

[42] Eek MN, Tranberg R, Zugner R, Alkema K, Beckung E. Muscle strength training to improve gait function in children with cerebral palsy. Dev Med Child Neurol. 2008;50(10):759–64.

[43] Taylor NF, Dodd KJ, Damiano DL. Progressive resistance exercise in physical therapy: a summary of systematic reviews. Phys Ther. 2005;85:1208–23.

[44] Lee JH, Sung IY, Yoo JY. Therapeutic effects of strengthening exercise on gait function of cerebral palsy. Disabil Rehabil. 2008;30(19):1439–44.

[45] Dodd KJ, Taylor NF, Graham HK. A randomized clinical trial of strength training in young people with cerebral palsy. Dev Med Child Neurol. 2003;45(10):652–7.

[46] Liao HF, Liu YC, Liu WY, Lin YT. Effectiveness of loaded sit-to-stand resistance exercise for children with mild spastic diplegia: a randomized clinical trial. Arch Phys Med Rehabil. 2007;88:25–31.

[47] Scholtes VA, Becher JG, Comuth A, Dekkers H, Van Dijk L, Dallmeijer AJ. Effectiveness of functional progressive resistance exercise strength training on muscle strength and mobility in children with cerebral palsy: a randomized controlled trial. Dev Med Child Neurol. 2010;52(6):e107–13.

[48] McCubbin AF, Shasby GB. Effects of isokinetic exercise on adolescents with cerebral palsy. Adapt Phys Activity Quart. 1985;2:56–64.

[49] Sherman W, Pearson D, Plyley M, Costill D, Habansky A, Vogelgesang D. Isokinetic rehabilitation after surgery. Am J Sports Med. 1982;10:155–61.

[50] Faigenbaum AD, Kraemer WJ, Blimkie CJ, Jeffreys I, Micheli LJ, Nitka M, et al. Youth resistance training: Updated position statement paper from the national strength and conditioning association. J Strength Cond Res. 2009;23:60–79.

[51] Anttila H, Autti-Ramo I, Suoranta J, Makela M, Malmivaara A. Effectiveness of physical therapy interventions for children with cerebral palsy: a systematic review. BMC Pediatr. 2008;8:14.

[52] Mockford M, Caulton JM. Systematic review of progressive strength training in children and adolescents with cerebral palsy who are ambulatory. Pediatr Phys Ther. 2008;20(4):318–33.

[53] Faigenbaum AD, Westcott WL, Micheli LJ, et al. The effects of strength training and detraining on children. J Strength Cond Res. 1996;10:109–14.

[54] Fowler EG, Kolobe TH, Damiano DL, et al. Promotion of physical fitness and prevention of secondary conditions for children with cerebral palsy: section on pediatrics research summit proceedings. Phys Ther. 2007;87:1495–510.

[55] Shortland A. Muscle deficits in cerebral palsy and early loss of mobility: can we learn something from our elders? Dev Med Child Neurol. 2009;51(4):59–63.

[56] Scholtes VA, Becher JG, Janssen-Potten YJ, Dekkers H, Smallenbroek L, Dallmeijer AJ. Effectiveness of functional progressive resistance exercise training on walking ability in children with cerebral palsy: a randomized controlled trial. Res Dev Disabil. 2012;33(1):181–8.

[57] Damiano DL, Dodd K, Taylor NF. Should we be testing and training muscle strength in cerebral palsy. Dev Med Child Neurol. 2002;44:68–72.

[58] Fowler EG, Knutson LM, DeMuth SK, Sugi M, Siebert K, Simms V, et al. Pediatric endurance and limb strengthening for children with cerebral palsy (PEDALS)–a randomized controlled trial protocol for a stationary cycling intervention. BMC Pediatr. 2007;7:14.

[59] Gregor R, Fowler EG. Biomechanics of cycling. In: Zachazewski J, Magee D, Quillen W, editors. Athletic Injuries and Rehabilitation. Philadelphia: W.B. Saunders Company; 1996. p. 367–88.

[60] Willoughby KL, Dodd KJ, Shields N. A systematic review of the effectiveness of treadmill training for children with cerebral palsy. Disabil Rehabil. 2009;31(24):1971–9.

[61] Mutlu A, Krosschell K, Spira DG. Treadmill training with partial body-weight support in children with cerebral palsy: a systematic review. Dev Med Child Neurol. 2009;51:260–75.

[62] Provost B, Dieruf K, Burtner PA, et al. Endurance and gait in children with cerebral palsy after intensive body weight-supported treadmill training. Pediatr Phys Ther. 2007;19:2–10.

[63] Dodd KJ, Foley S. Partial body-weight-supported treadmill training can improve walking in children with cerebral palsy: a clinical controlled trial. Dev Med Child Neurol. 2007;49:101–5.

[64] Damiano DL, DeJong SL. A systematic review of the effectiveness of treadmill training and body weight support in pediatric rehabilitation. J Neurol Phys Ther. 2009;33(1):27–44.

[65] Richards C, Malouin F, Dumas F, Marcoux S, Lepage C, Menier C. Early and intensive treadmill locomotor training for young children with cerebral palsy: a feasibility study. Pediatr Phys Ther. 1997;9:158–65.

[66] Damiano D. Strengthening exercises. In: Miller F, editor. Physical Therapy for Cerebral Palsy. Wilmington: Springer; 2007. p. 346–8.

[67] Braendvik SM, Elvrum AK, Vereijken B, Roeleveld K. Involuntary and voluntary muscle activation in children with unilateral cerebral palsy – Relationship to upper limb activity. Eur J Paediatr Neurol. 2013;17(3):274–9.

[68] Braendvik SM, Roeleveld K. The role of co-activation in strength and force modulation in the elbow of children with unilateral cerebral palsy. J Electromyogr Kinesiol. 2012;22(1):137–44.

[69] Smits-Engelsman BC, Rameckers EA, Duysens J. Muscle force generation and force control of finger movements in children with spastic hemiplegia during isometric tasks. Dev Med Child Neurol. 2005;47(5):337–42.

[70] Elvrum AK, Braendvik SM, Saether R, Lamvik T, Vereijken B, Roeleveld K. Effectiveness of resistance training in combination with botulinum toxin-A on hand and arm use in children with cerebral palsy: A pre-post intervention study. BMC Pediatrics. 2012;12:91.

[71] Kamper DG, Yasukawa AM, Barrett KM, Gaebler-Spira DJ. Effects of neuromuscular electrical stimulation treatment of cerebral palsy on potential impairment mechanisms: a pilot study. Pediatr Phys Ther. 2006;18(1):31–8.

[72] Franki I, Desloovere K, De Cat J, Feys H, Molenaers G, Calders P, et al. The evidence-base for conceptual approaches and additional therapies targeting lower limb function in children with cerebral palsy: a systematic review using the ICF as a framework. J Rehabil Med. 2012;44(5):396–405.

[73] Rameckers EA, Duysens J, Speth LA, Vles HJ, Smits-Engelsman BC. Effect of addition of botulinum toxin-A to standardized therapy for dynamic manual skills measured with kinematic aiming tasks in children with spastic hemiplegia. J Rehabil Med. 2010;42(4):332–8.

[74] Kim DA, Lee JA, Hwang PW, Lee MJ, Kim HK, Park JJ, et al. The effect of comprehensive hand repetitive intensive strength training (CHRIST) using motion analysis in children with cerebral palsy. Ann Rehabil Med. 2012;36(1):39–46.

[75] Kelly M, Darrah J. Aquatic exercise for children with cerebral palsy. Dev Med Child Neurol. 2005;47(12):838–42.

[76] Fragala-Pinkham M, Haley SM, O'neil ME. Group aquatic aerobic exercise for children with disabilities. Dev Med Child Neurol. 2008;50(11):822–827.

[77] Fragala-Pinkham MA, Dumas HM, Barlow CA, Pasternak A. An aquatic physical therapy program at a pediatric rehabilitation hospital: a case series. Pediatr Phys Ther. 2009;21(1):68–78.

[78] Verschuren O, Ketelaar M, Takken T, Helders PJM, Gorter JW. Exercise programs for children with cerebral palsy: a systematic review of the literature. Am J Phys Med Rehabil. 2008;87(5):404–17.

[79] Becker BE. Aquatic therapy: scientific foundations and clinical rehabilitation applications. PM&R. 2009;1(9):859–72.

[80] Brunton LK, Bartlett DJ. Description of exercise participation of adolescents with cerebral palsy across a 4-year period. Pediatr Phys Ther. 2010;22(2):180–7.

[81] Zwier JN, Van Schie PEM, Becher JG, Smits DW, Gorter JW, Dallmeijer AJ. Physical activity in young children with cerebral palsy. Dis Rehabil. 2010;32(18):1501–8.

[82] Zick CD, Smith KR, Brown BB, Fan JX, Kowaleski-Jones L. Physical activity during the transition from adolescence to adulthood. J Phys Act Health. 2007;4:125–37.

[83] Kemper CG. The Amsterdam Growth Study: A Longitudinal Analysis of Health, Fitness, and Lifestyle. Champaign, IL: Human Kinetics; 1995.

[84] King G, Law M, King S, Rosenbaum P, Kertoy MK, Young NL. A conceptual model of the factors affecting the recreation and leisure participation of children with disabilities. Phys Occup Ther Pediatr. 2003;23:63–90.

[85] Burgeson CR, Wechsler H, Brener ND, Young JC, Spain CG. Physical education and activity: results from the School Health Policies and Programs Study. J Sch Health. 2001;71:279–93.

[86] Murphy N, Carbone P. Council on children with disabilities. Promoting the participation of children with disabilities in sports, recreation, and physical activities. Pediatrics. 2008;121(5):1057–61.

[87] Grunbaum JA, Kann L, Kinchen SA, Williams B, Ross JE, Lowery R, Kolbe L. Youth risk behavior surveillance-United States, 2001. MMWR Surveill Summ. 2002;51:1–61.

[88] Fernhall B, Unnithan VB. Physical activity, metabolic issues, and assessment. Phys Med Rehabil Clin N Am. 2002;13:925–47.

[89] Kerr C, McDowell B, McDonough S. Electrical stimulation in cerebral palsy: a review of effects on strength and motor function. Dev Med Child Neurol. 2004;46(3):205–13.

[90] Fırat T, Ayhan Ç, Meriç A, Kırdı N. Çocuklarda Elektroterapi Uygulamaları. Turkiye Klinikleri J PM&R-Special Topics. 2010;3(3):101–6.

[91] Chiu HC, Ada L. Effect of functional electrical stimulation on activity in children with cerebral palsy: a systematic review. Pediatr Phys Ther. 2014;26(3):283–8.

[92] Reed B. The physiology of neuromuscular electrical stimulation. Pediatr Phys Ther. 1997;9:96–102.

[93] Kapadia NM, Nagai MK, Zivanovic V, Bernstein J, Woodhouse J, Rumney P, et al. Functional electrical stimulation therapy for recovery of reaching and grasping in severe chronic pediatric stroke patients. J Child Neurol. 2014;29(4):493–9.

[94] Pieber K, Herceg M, Wick F, Grim-Stieger M, Bernert G, Paternostro-Sluga T. Functional electrical stimulation combined with botulinum toxin type A to improve hand function in children with spastic hemiparesis—a pilot study. Wien Klin Wochenschr. 2011;123(3–4):100–5.

[95] Scheffler LR, Chae J. Neuromuscular electrical stimulation in neurorehabilitation. Muscle Nerve. 2007;35:562–90.

[96] Hamzaid NA, Pithon KR, Smith RM, Davis GM. Functional electrical stimulation elliptical stepping versus cycling in spinal cord-injured individuals. Clin Biomech (Bristol, Avon). 2012;27(7):731–7.

[97] Franki I, Desloovere K, De Cat J, Feys H, Molenaers G, Calders P, et al. The evidence-base for basic physical therapy techniques targeting lower limb function in children with cerebral palsy: a systematic review using the International Classification of Functioning, Disability and Health as a conceptual framework. J Rehabil Med. 2012;44:385–95.

[98] Stackhouse SK, Binder-Macleod SA, Stackhouse CA, McCarthy JJ, Prosser LA, Lee SC. Neuromuscular electrical stimulation versus volitional isometric strength training in children with spastic diplegic cerebral palsy: a preliminary study. Neurorehabil Neural Repair. 2007;21(6):475–85.

[99] Pape KE. Therapeutic electrical stimulation (TES) for the treatment of disuse muscle atrophy in cerebral palsy. Pediatr Phys Ther. 1997;9:110–2.

[100] Sommerfelt K, Markestad T, Berg K, Saetesdal I. Therapeutic electrical stimulation in cerebral palsy: a randomized, controlled, crossover trial. Dev Med Child Neurol. 2001;43(9):609–13.

[101] Dali C, Hansen FJ, Pedersen SA, Skov L, Hilden J, Bjornskov I, et al. Threshold electrical stimulation (TES) in ambulant children with CP: a randomized double-blind placebo-controlled clinical trial. Dev Med Child Neurol. 2002;44(6):364–9.

[102] Maenpaa H, Jaakkola R, Sandstrom M, von Wendt L. Effect of sensory-level electrical stimulation of the tibialis anterior muscle during physical therapy on active dorsiflexion of the ankle of children with cerebral palsy. Pediatr Phys Ther. 2004;16(1):39–44.

[103] Mayston M. The Bobath concept-evolution and application. In: Forssberg H, Hirschfeld H, editors. Movement Disorders in Children. Basel: Krager; 1992. p. 1–6.

[104] Damiano DL, Abel MF. Functional outcomes of strength training in spastic cerebral palsy. Arch Phys Med Rehabil. 1998;79(2):119–25.

[105] Darrah J, Wessel J, Nearingburg P, O'Connor M. Evaluation of a community fitness program for adolescents with cerebral palsy. Pediatr Phys Ther. 1999;11:18–23.

[106] Lockwood RJ. Effects of Isokinetic Strength Training on Strength and Motor Skill in Athletes with Cerebral Palsy. Perth, Australia: Australian Sports Commission; 1993.

Section 4

Interventions

Chapter 6

Orthodontic Treatment in Children with Cerebral Palsy

María Teresa Abeleira, Mercedes Outumuro,
Marcio Diniz, Lucía García-Caballero, Pedro Diz and
Jacobo Limeres

Additional information is available at the end of the chapter

http://dx.doi.org/10.5772/64639

Abstract

Cerebral palsy is a permanent neuromuscular motor disorder that gives rise to many functional problems, including impaired swallowing, chewing and speech. Maxillary transverse deficiency and Angle Class II malocclusion are common. Some of these functional problems can be due to maxillary malocclusion. To our knowledge, no case series has yet been published on orthodontic treatment in children with cerebral palsy. In this chapter, we provide an overview of this topic based on the literature and on our own clinical experience. We consider that some patients with cerebral palsy are susceptible to orthodontic treatment. The keys to success are appropriate patient selection, based on anatomical, physiological and behavioural characteristics, and the degree of involvement of parents and caregivers. Among parents of cerebral palsy children undergoing orthodontic therapy, the perceived level of overall satisfaction was very high and expectations were often exceeded; however, these results are conditioned by factors such as the Peer Assessment Rating (PAR) index. Although some authors reported improvements in aesthetics, speech and oral function, an objective assessment of functional improvement is still lacking. In our experience, correction of resting position and management of neuromuscular alterations are essential if successful orthodontic treatment is to be achieved and relapses avoided.

Keywords: cerebral palsy, malocclusion, orthodontic treatment, oral function, special care dentistry

1. Introduction

Cerebral palsy (CP) carries a significant morbidity and has a limited life expectancy [1]. We should therefore ask ourselves the following question: Are these patients susceptible to orthodontic treatment? The main indication for orthodontic treatment is dental malocclusion. In 1956, Lyons [2] had already suggested that CP had effects on dentofacial development and, in particular, on tooth occlusion (to facilitate comprehension, a glossary of orthodontic terms has been included at the end of the chapter [**Box 1**]). The most common malocclusions described in CP patients are overjet and overbite, which have significantly higher prevalences in these patients than in healthy controls matched for sex and race [3]. Overjet ≥ 4 mm has been reported in around 70% of spastic CP children and anterior open bite ≥ 2 mm in up to 90% of cases [4]. Compared with other physical disabilities, there is a particularly high prevalence of open bite in CP; it is estimated that children diagnosed with CP have a threefold greater chance of having open bite than children with other special needs [5]. Paradoxically, when anteroposterior malocclusion is analysed, the prevalence of Angle Class I (normo-occlusion) in patients with CP is higher than in the general population [3]. However, malocclusion in the vertical plane provokes marked functional alterations that, in some cases, could justify performing orthopaedic-orthodontic treatment (**Figure 1**).

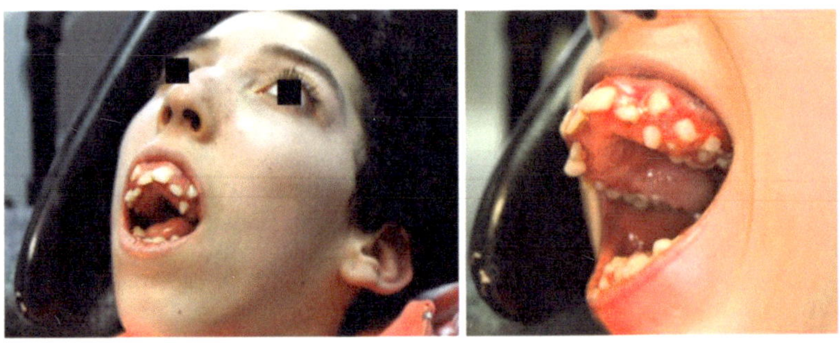

Figure 1. Severe open bite and oral functional impairment in a spastic cerebral palsy patient.

2. Severity of malocclusion

A study carried out in Minas Gerais in Brazil, with the participation of 60 spastic CP children and 60 age-matched controls, showed that some orofacial alterations with functional repercussions were more common in CP children than in the controls: severe lip incompetence was 2.8 times more common, mouth breathing 4.8 times more common and long facies 5.4 times more common [4]. Unfortunately, oral functionality is often left as a secondary issue when discussing the need for orthodontic treatment and many dental practitioners focus treatment on cosmetic objectives. The index most widely used for this purpose is the Dental Aesthetic Index (DAI), published 30 years ago by investigators in the University of Iowa. That index gives us the following classification for malocclusion: mild or absent (DAI score <25), defined (DAI = 26–30), severe (DAI = 31–35) and very severe or debilitating (DAI > 35) [6]. 'Severe' and 'very severe' malocclusions (DAI ≥ 31) are usually considered susceptible to orthodontic correction from a cosmetic point of view [6]. In a study of 44 CP patients of 12–59 years of age performed in Spain, significant differences were observed in the DAI scores for lip incompetence and mouth breathing compared with healthy controls [7]. In that series, resting head position also affected the DAI score; the highest scores were observed in patients with absent resting heading position control, followed by those who held their head permanently in flexion, those who held their head in hyperextension and, finally, those with a resting head position in a vertical axis [7].

A relevant issue is whether CP patients with associated mental disability have a less favourable facial phenotype than those with an intellectual coefficient in the normal range (**Figure 2**). On this subject, a study performed in Leeds, in the United Kingdom, found significantly greater overjet in CP with mental disability (mean of 8.3 versus 5.5 mm) as well as a higher frequency of Angle Class II division 1 (Class II-1) malocclusion (75% versus 36%) [3].

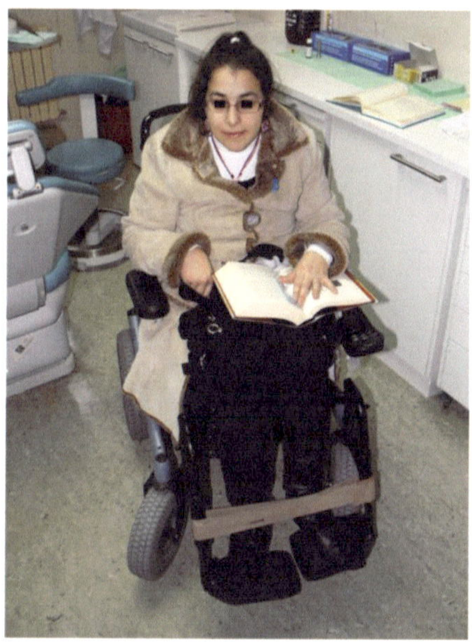

Figure 2. Cerebral palsy is a physical disability and many patients have a normal intelligence.

3. Orthodontic management

No large series of CP patients undergoing orthodontic treatment has been published in the literature, with the exception of a group of 62 adult CP individuals living in Bad Oeynhausen in Bielefeld, Germany; 32% of the patients aged between 18 and 36 years had worn orthodontic appliances, whereas none of the 31 patients aged over 36 years had received treatment. A possible interpretation of such a difference is that it could have been due to the individual initiative of a single dental practitioner or group of practitioners, and the results should therefore be extrapolated with a degree of caution [8]. It has been suggested that the aims of orthodontic treatment in patients with disabilities should focus on optimal aesthetic improvement and enhanced social acceptance, taking into account that an 'ideal' treatment may not be possible [9]. In a review of the literature, we found no studies or case reports that explored the benefits and effects of functional or fixed orthodontic appliance therapy in children with CP [10].

The following basic requirements need to be satisfied when considering orthodontic treatment in children with disabilities: the commitment of the patient and of the parents/carers, adequate oral hygiene, the degree of patient collaboration (behaviour management) and manual dexterity [11]. The criteria for patient selection are detailed in **Table 1**.

• Medical condition
• Malocclusion
• Aesthetic assessment
• Parent/carer commitment
• Child's tolerance to treatment
• Oral hygiene
• Risk/benefit ratio

Table 1. Selection criteria for patients with severe disabilities who are candidates for orthodontic treatment (modified from [9]).

• Impressions using quick-set materials
• Easy bonding of brackets
• Self-etching primer
• Advanced memory wires
• Self-ligating brackets
• Oral functionality
• Advances in orthognathic surgery
• Reversible mini-implant anchorage

Table 2. Technological innovations for dental patients with disabilities (modified with permission from Becker and Shapira [11]).

Certain technological improvements in dentistry in recent years could benefit disabled dental patients in general, including CP patients receiving orthodontic treatment [12] (**Table 2**). These technical innovations and the creation of multidisciplinary teams have made it possible to undertake orthodontic treatment in CP patients with extra-oral appliances (**Figure 3**), fixed multi-bracket appliances (**Figure 4**) and even complex orthodontic treatments and orthognathic surgery (**Figure 5**).

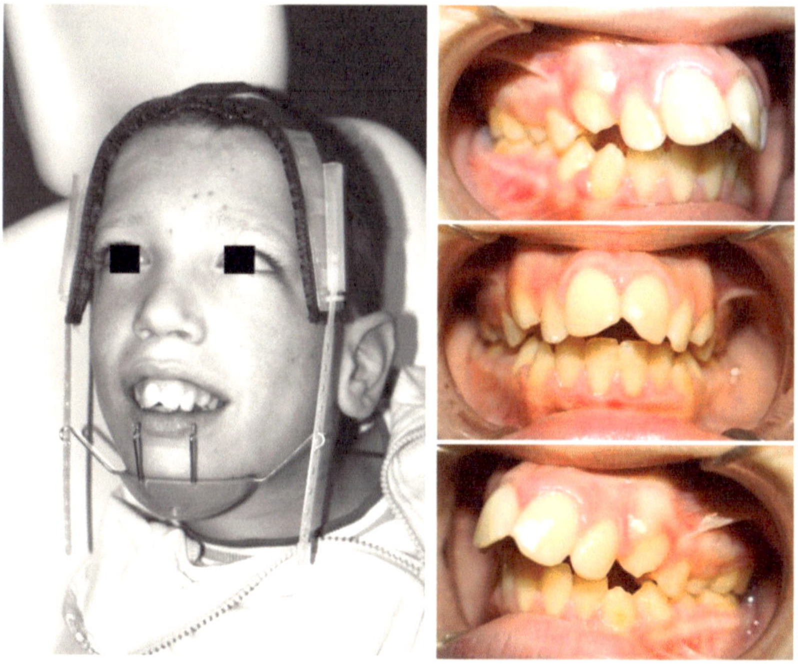

Figure 3. Cerebral palsy patient with severe Class II-1 malocclusion. Initial phase of orthodontic treatment with a face mask.

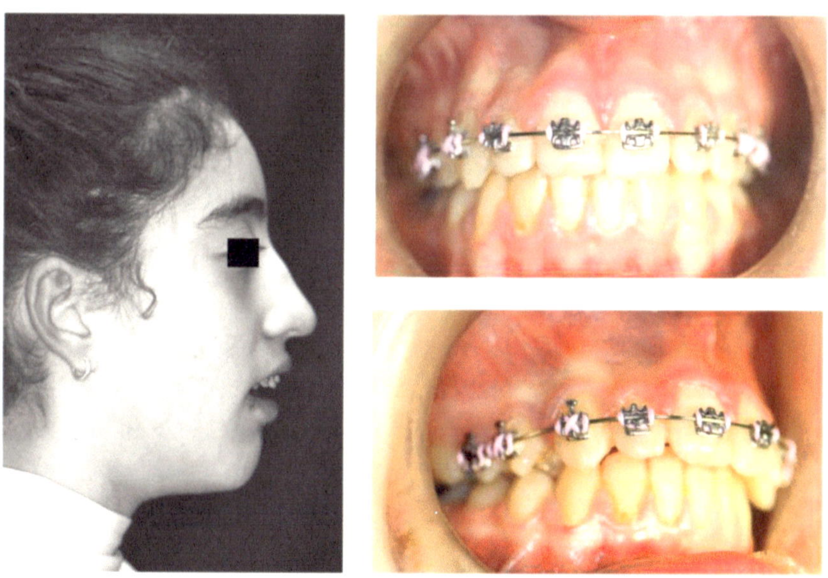

Figure 4. Cerebral palsy patient with Class II-1 malocclusion treated with fixed multi-bracket appliances.

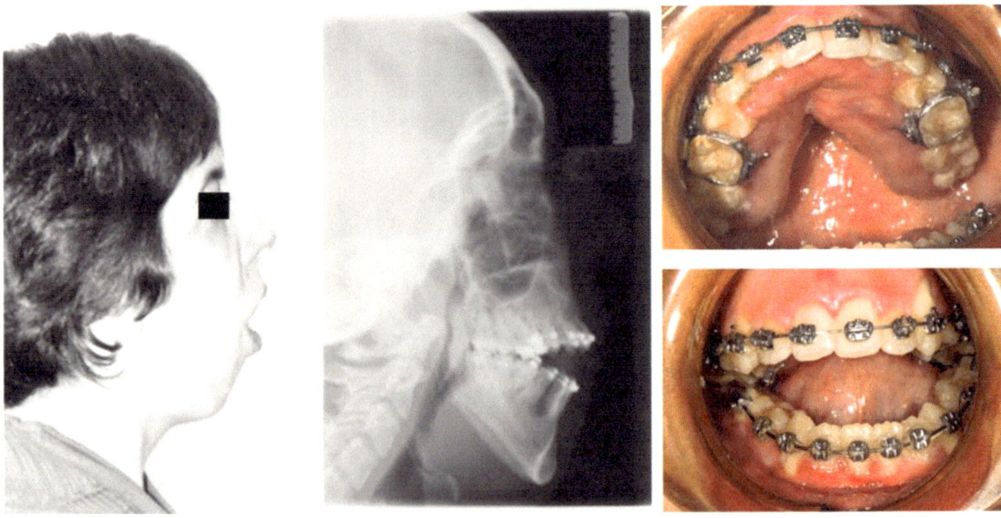

Figure 5. Cerebral palsy patient with open bite treated using fixed multi-bracket appliances before undergoing orthognathic surgery.

4. Identifying success criteria

Evaluation of the results of orthodontic treatment as successful or unsuccessful requires more than simply quantifying the aesthetic improvement. Parameters such as oral functionality, quality of life and, very importantly, relapse rates must also be taken into account.

In 2014, İşcan et al. [10] published a case report of a 12-year-old girl with ataxic CP who had Class II malocclusion, maxillary transverse deficiency and severe crowding. Treatment consisted of maxillary expansion with simultaneous functional therapy, fixed multi-bracket appliances and a vertical chin cup. The authors reported that acceptable occlusion, improvements in swallowing, speech and drooling, better masticatory muscle activity and a reduction in problems of impaired chewing were achieved [10]. That study demonstrated the need to develop tools able to quantify oral functional deficits—similar to the tools used to quantify cosmetic appearance, such as the Dental Aesthetic Index—to provide an objective assessment of the functional improvements accomplished by orthodontic treatment.

A survey of satisfaction and the appreciation of improvements answered by the parents of disabled children—including CP children—who underwent orthodontic treatment made the following findings: results exceeded expectations in 42% of cases, the reaction of friends and relatives was defined as 'they got excited' in 54% of cases, there was a very marked improvement in patient daily activities in 81% of cases, and the child's social life improved significantly according to 45% of respondents [13]. An analysis of the benefits of orthodontic treatment as perceived by the parents of disabled children reported that improvement in quality of life was a response given by 83% of surveyed parents, improvement in social acceptance in 78% of cases and improvement in social integration in 71% of cases. Interestingly, when asked about their desire to enhance dental and facial appearance, only 68% of participants answered 'a lot' and 20% 'a little' [13].

We have found no published studies designed specifically to address the issue of improvement in the quality of life of CP children following orthodontic treatment. In a study performed in Sao Paulo, Brazil, in which the parents of 60 CP children aged 6–14 years were interviewed, it was found that the Child Oral Health-Related Quality of Life Questionnaire (COHRQoL) score was not affected by the presence of malocclusion, dental injuries or dental fluorosis, but, in contrast, there was a significant correlation with a history of dental caries, bruxism and family income [14].

5. Follow-up and relapse prevention

Regular dental check-ups are mandatory in patients with CP because they are more prone to oral health problems related to enamel hypoplasia, pasty food intake, difficulty in maintaining good oral hygiene, drug-induced gingival hyperplasia and periodontal disease [4]. Consequently, parents and caregivers have to receive oral hygiene and diet instructions to avoid carious lesions, and patient will receive professional scaling at regular intervals before, during and after orthodontic treatment, to avoid periodontal disease [15].

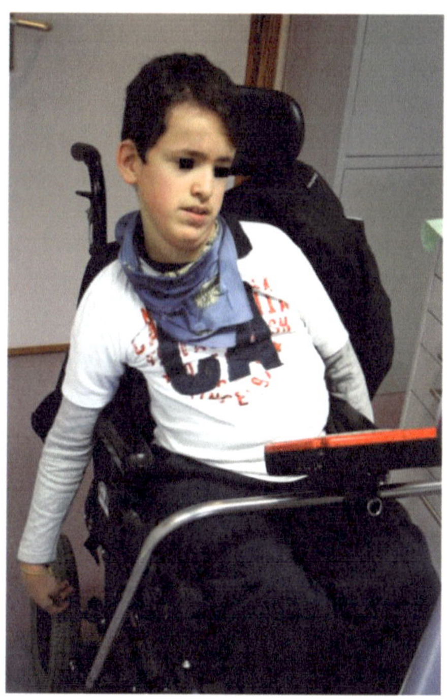

Figure 6. Cerebral palsy patient with severe scoliosis that altered the resting position and affected the occlusal pattern (unilateral open bite).

In an article published in 1927 by Stillwell [16], it was suggested that malocclusion and scoliosis affected posture and that this was a two-way relationship, in that alterations of posture also had repercussions on the teeth and the spine. This factor is probably often underestimated by health professionals, and it needs to be taken into account to be able to assess the risk of relapse. The relationship between malocclusion and vertebral alignment was demonstrated in an experimental model in animals (rats), in which the application of resin to induce unilateral premature tooth contact provoked iatrogenic scoliosis within a few weeks; this alteration was reversible when natural occlusal contact was restored [17]. This relationship is so strong that it has been suggested that the detection of hereditary malocclusions in young children 'allows the identification of a group of children who have a high risk of developing scoliosis in later years' [18]. In a systematic review published in 2011, it was concluded that there is plausible evidence for an increased prevalence of unilateral Angle Class II malocclusions associated with scoliosis and an increased risk of lateral crossbite and midline deviation in children affected by scoliosis [19] (**Figure 6**).

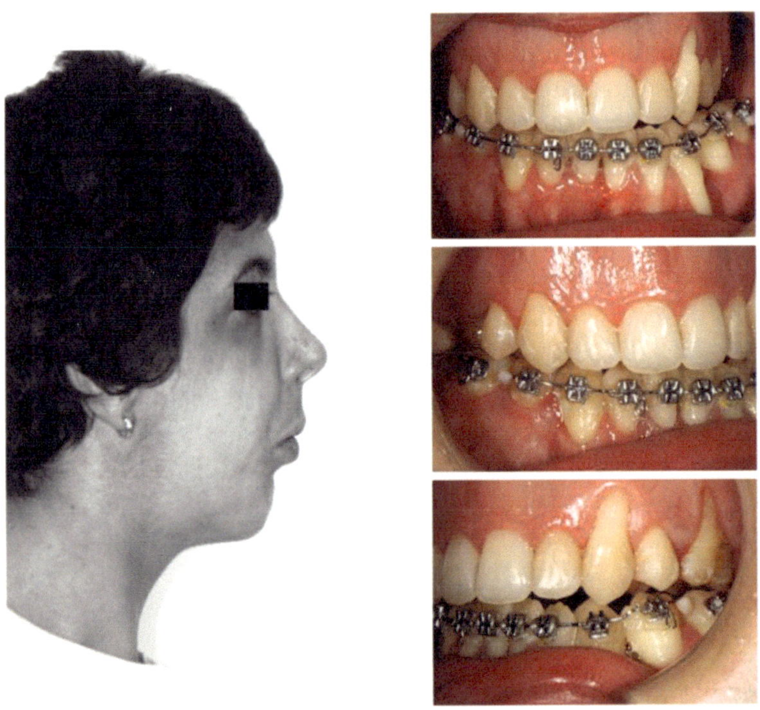

Figure 7. Cerebral palsy patient with open bite relapse after treatment with fixed multi-bracket appliances and orthognathic surgery.

Although the routine use of specific braces to stabilise the spine in CP children was initiated in the second half of the nineteenth century, certain improvements have been made to the modern versions of these braces. Probably the most popular model is the Milwaukee brace, whose effect on dentofacial growth has been described in detail, particularly with regard to

http://dx.doi.org/10.5772/64639

abnormal proclination of the upper and lower incisor teeth [20]. Descriptions of cases of orthodontic treatment for malocclusion associated with scoliosis (mainly overjet) have also been published [21].

All these contributions indirectly confirm not only the close two-way relationship between resting position and malocclusion but also introduce a new conditioning factor, neuromuscular alterations, particularly relevant when muscle hypertonicity or spasticity is present. In our experience, these three factors are the principal determinants of relapse, and orthodontic treatment in patients with CP should not be initiated without first evaluating muscle tone and resting position. To illustrate this proposal, we only have to look at the case described by İşcan et al. [10] that we commented above. Their patient presented a certain degree of unilateral posterior open bite in the follow-up photographs. Relapse, even if less severe than the initial occlusal situation, can overshadow the success of a complex treatment, such as in the patient shown in **Figure 5**. After prolonged orthodontic treatment with fixed multi-bracket appliances and bimaxillary orthognathic surgery, that patient developed a relapse with unilateral open bite and marked gingival retraction secondary to muscle hypertonicity (**Figure 7**).

Spasticity of masseter and temporalis muscles causes hypertonia—spastic hypertonia—that aggravates the mandibular malposition (mandible is usually located in a retrograde and posteriorly rotated position) and may promote relapses after orthodontic treatment. It has been shown that intramuscularly injected botulinum toxin type A significantly decreases muscle spasticity [22], which hypothetically may help to prevent relapse in selected cases.

6. Conclusions

Orthodontic treatment is feasible in CP children after careful patient selection, taking into account that success depends not only on obvious factors, such as the type and severity of malocclusion and the degree of patient collaboration, but also on resting position and neuromuscular disturbances. The objective assessment of treatment success requires the application of tools that quantitatively evaluate improvements in the domains of aesthetic appearance, oral functionality and quality of life. Unconventional treatment plans have to be chosen at times, and parents must be thoroughly informed to avoid inappropriate expectations.

Box 1. Glossary of orthodontic terms

Angle's classification system: A method used to classify different types of malocclusion, based on the mesiodistal relationship of the permanent molars on their eruption and locking.

Bracket: A metal, plastic or ceramic element that is glued onto a tooth and that holds a metal wire called an arch wire; this system produces or guides orthodontic tooth movement.

Class I: A malocclusion where the upper teeth line up with your bottom teeth (but the teeth are crooked, crowded or turned).

Class II: A malocclusion where the upper teeth protrude beyond the lower teeth. This is also called 'overbite' or 'buck teeth'.

Class III: A malocclusion in which the lower teeth protrude beyond the upper teeth.

Crossbite: A malocclusion in which some of the upper teeth are inside of the lower teeth when the jaws are closed.

Crowding: An orthodontic problem caused by insufficient space for the teeth.

Fixed appliance: An orthodontic component that is cemented or bonded to the teeth.

Malocclusion: A poor alignment of the upper and lower teeth in the anteroposterior or transverse planes when the jaws are closed.

Overjet: An extension of the incisal or buccal cusp ridges of the upper teeth horizontally (labially or buccally) beyond the ridges of the lower teeth when the jaws are closed normally.

Overbite: An extension of the incisal ridges of the upper anterior teeth below the incisal ridges of the corresponding lower teeth when the jaws are closed normally.

Open bite: A malocclusion that occurs in the vertical plane, characterized by lack of vertical overlap between the maxillary and mandibular dentition.

Self-ligating brackets: Ligatureless bracket systems that have a mechanical device built into the bracket to close off the edgewise slot.

Author details

María Teresa Abeleira, Mercedes Outumuro, Marcio Diniz, Lucía García-Caballero, Pedro Diz* and Jacobo Limeres

*Address all correspondence to: pedro.diz@usc.es

Special Needs Unit and OMEQUI Research Group, School of Medicine and Dentistry, Santiago de Compostela University, Santiago de Compostela, Galicia, Spain

References

[1] Himmelmann, K., Sundh, V. (2015). Survival with cerebral palsy over five decades in western Sweden. *Developmental Medicine & Child Neurology*, 57(8), 762–767.

http://dx.doi.org/10.5772/64639

[2] Lyons, D.C. (1956). An evaluation of the effects of cerebral palsy on dentofacial development, especially occlusion of the teeth. *Journal of Pediatrics*, 49(4), 432–436.

[3] Franklin, D.L., Luther,F., Curzon, M.E. (1996). The prevalence of malocclusion in children with cerebral palsy. *European Journal of Orthodontics*, 18(6), 637–643.

[4] Miamoto, C.B., Ramos-Jorge, M.L., Pereira, L.J., Paiva, S.M., Pordeus, I.A., Marques, L.S. (2010). Severity of malocclusion in patients with cerebral palsy: determinant factors. *The American Journal of Orthodontics and Dentofacial Orthopedics*, 138(394), e1–e5.

[5] Oliveira, A.C., Paiva, S.M., Martins, M.T., Torres, C.S., Pordeus, I.A. (2011). Prevalence and determinant factors of malocclusion in children with special needs. *European Journal of Orthodontics*, 33(4), 413–418.

[6] Cons, N.C., Jenny, J., Kohout, F.J. (1986). DAI: The Dental Aesthetic Index. Iowa City, Iowa: College of Dentistry, University of Iowa.

[7] Martinez-Mihi, V., Silvestre, F.J., Orellana, L.M., Silvestre-Rangil, J. (2014). Resting position of the head and malocclusion in a group of patients with cerebral palsy. *Journal of Clinical and Experimental Dentistry*, 6(1), e1–e6.

[8] Asdaghi Mamaghani, S.M., Bode, H., Ehmer, U. (2008). Orofacial findings in conjunction with infantile cerebral paralysis in adults of two different age groups a cross-sectional study. *Journal of Orofacial Orthopedics*, 69(4), 240–256.

[9] Chadwick, S.M., Asher-Mcdade, C. (1997). The orthodontic management of patients with profound learning disability. *British Journal of Orthodontics*, 24(2), 117–125.

[10] İşcan, H.N., Metin-Gürsoy, G., Kale-Varlik, S. (2014). Functional and fixed orthodontic treatment in a child with cerebral palsy. *The American Journal of Orthodontics and Dentofacial Orthopedics*, 145(4), 523–533.

[11] Becker, A., Shapira, J. (1996). Orthodontics for the handicapped child. *European Journal of Orthodontics*, 18(1), 55–67.

[12] Musich, D.R. (2006). Orthodontic intervention and patients with Down syndrome. *The Angle Orthodontist*, 76(4), 734–735.

[13] Abeleira, M.T., Pazos, E., Ramos, I., Outumuro, M., Limeres, J., Seoane-Romero, J., Diniz, M., Diz, P. (2014). Orthodontic treatment for disabled children: a survey of parents' attitudes and overall satisfaction. *BMC Oral Health*, 14, 98.

[14] Abanto, J., Ortega, A.O.L., Raggio D.P., Bönecker M., Mendes F.M., Ciamponi A.L. (2014). Impact of oral diseases and disorders on oral-health-related quality of life of children with cerebral palsy. *Special Care in Dentistry*, 34(2), 56–63.

[15] Sabuncuoglu, F.A., Özcan, E. (2014). Orthodontic management of a patient with cerebral palsy: six years follow-up. *Journal of Contemporary Dental Practice*, 15(4), 491–495.

[16] Stillwell, F.S. (1927). The correlation of malocclusion and scoliosis to posture and its effect upon the teeth and spine. *Dental Cosmos*, 69, 154–163.

[17] D′Attilio, M., Filippi, M.R., Femminella, B., Festa, F., Tecco, S. (2005). The influence of an experimentally-induced malocclusion on vertebral alignment in rats: a controlled pilot study. *Cranio*, 23(2), 119–129.

[18] Pećina, M., Lulić-Dukić, O., Pećina-Hrncević, A. (1991). Hereditary orthodontic anomalies and idiopathic scoliosis. *International Orthopedics*, 15(1), 57–59.

[19] Saccucci, M., Tettamanti, L., Mummolo, S., Polimeni, A., Festa, F., Tecco, S. (2011). Scoliosis and dental occlusion: a review of the literature. *Scoliosis*, 6, 15.

[20] Rock, W.P., Baker, R. (1972). The effect of the Milwaukee brace upon dentofacial growth. *The Angle Orthodontist*, 42(2), 96–102.

[21] Hitchcock, H.P. (1969). Treatment of a malocclusion associated with scoliosis. *The Angle Orthodontist*, 39(1), 64–68.

[22] Manzano, F.S., Granero, L.M., Masiero, D., dos, Maria, TB. (2004). Treatment of muscle spasticity in patients with cerebral palsy using BTX-A: a pilot study. *Special Care in Dentistry*, 24(4), 235–239.

Chapter 7

Neuromusculoskeletal Rehabilitation of Severe Cerebral Palsy

Deepak Sharan, Joshua Samuel Rajkumar,
Rajarajeshwari Balakrishnan and Amruta Kulkarni

Additional information is available at the end of the chapter

http://dx.doi.org/10.5772/64642

Abstract

Persons with Gross Motor Function Classification System (GMFCS) levels IV and V are considered as severe cerebral palsy (CP) and are non-ambulatory. These persons are at a higher risk of complications such as hip displacement (sub-luxation or dislocation), spinopelvic deformities, musculoskeletal pain, low bone mineral density and low energy fracture. The recommended management strategy at present for this group is wheelchair-aided mobility, with which none of these complications can be prevented. There is a strong need to evaluate alternative methods of treatment that can allow assisted ambulation in persons with severe CP. The role of Single Event Multilevel Lever Arm Restoration and AntiSpasticity Surgery (SEMLARASS) and protocol-based active rehabilitation on gross motor function and ambulation of non-ambulatory persons with CP at GMFCS levels IV and V is examined. Active rehabilitation involves making the person with severe CP active through most of the waking hours and participating actively in the rehabilitation. A well-planned and executed SEMLARASS, followed by intensive, protocol-based, sequenced multidisciplinary active rehabilitation, provides the persons with GMFCS levels IV and V a significant functional improvement in gross motor function and mobility.

Keywords: cerebral palsy, neuromusculoskeletal rehabilitation, SEMLARASS, active rehabilitation, GMFCS

1. Introduction

Cerebral palsy (CP) is a non-progressive disorder affecting the individual's posture, movement, and causing limitation in the activities that are permanent, caused due to damage in developing brain of neonates or infants. CP causes not only motor disturbances, but also sensory, cognitive, social, behaviour, speech and communication, seizure disorder, respiratory illness and other musculoskeletal disorders [1]. A total of 17 million persons are estimated to have CP worldwide and CP is one of the most common causes of physical disability among children. The prevalence of CP is currently estimated to be 2.11/1000 live births [2] and varies between 1 and 5/1000 live births in different countries. 28% of persons with CP have epilepsy, 58% have difficulties with communication, 42% have visual problems and 23–56% have learning disabilities [3].

Clinicians classify patients with CP to describe the specific problem, to predict prognosis and to guide treatment. Classification is based on the change in muscle tone, anatomical region of involvement and severity of the problem. Types of CP according to muscle tone are spastic (hemiplegia, diplegia and quadriplegia based on anatomical region of involvement), ataxic and dyskinetic (dystonia and choreoathetosis). Even though these terms do not have specific reliability among the observers, these terms are helpful for understanding the CP condition [4]. Gross Motor Function Classification System (GMFCS) is another system to classify gross motor function of children and youths with CP on the basis of their self-initiated movement with particular emphasis on sitting, walking and wheeled mobility. Children and youths with GMFCS levels IV and V are non-ambulatory and are considered as severe CP. Persons in GMFCS level IV use wheelchair, either manual or automatic, for transportation and persons in GMFCS level V are highly dependent because of the lack of balance in head, neck and trunk, and will require major assistive devices for physical assistance [5].

According to data from North India, 69% of persons with CP had spastic quadriplegia or dyskinetic CP and were non-ambulatory [6]. These persons are at a higher risk of developing complications such as hip displacement (sub-luxation or dislocation), spinopelvic deformities, musculoskeletal pain, low bone mineral density and low energy fracture. The most common and serious structural change in persons who have severe CP is hip displacement. This deformity is seldom present at birth but develops as the child grows older and experiences abnormal muscle pull from spastic muscles, increased femoral anteversion and the lack of weight bearing on the lower extremities. The reported rates of hip displacement in persons with CP vary from 1 to 75% [7]. The incidence of hip displacement in CP is related to the severity of involvement, varying from 1% in children with spastic hemiplegia up to 75% in those with spastic quadriplegia [8]. In two population studies, the rate of hip displacement was found to be one-third and was not related to the movement disorder but was directly related to gross motor function as determined by the GMFCS [9, 10].

The prevalence of hip pain in severe CP is reported to be 47.2% [11]. The common type of pain identified was provoked pain (e.g. during mobilisation, palpation and weight bearing on the lower extremities). A study of 2777 children (57% boys) at a median age of 7 years reported 32.4% children in pain, with significantly more girls than boys experiencing pain, and significantly more children at GMFCS levels III and V than GMFCS level I. The frequency of pain increased with age. Pain in the abdomen and hips was most frequent at GMFCS V, whereas knee pain was most frequent at level III and foot pain at level I [12].

Markedly low bone mass in children and adults with severe CP has been reported to place these persons at the risk of osteopenia, osteoporosis and low-energy fracture [13].

http://dx.doi.org/10.5772/64642

Increasing problems with reduced mobility lead to problems with daily activities especially in instrumental activities of daily living (IADL). Social participation, sexual relationships, employment and leisure activities are restricted among many youths and young adults with severe CP [14–18]. Severities of physical and/or cognitive impairment are predictors for limited participation, but limited participation is not necessarily synonymous with a poorer quality of life [14, 19, 20]. Some studies also show that pain, falling stamina and functional deterioration have a negative impact on the quality of life.

Several potential benefits exist for making a person with severe CP ambulate in a therapeutic setting:

1. The ability to retain standing transfers in adolescents and young adults with CP means that they do not require lifting or hoisting by their caregivers, thereby reducing the risk of musculoskeletal disorders in caregivers [21].
2. Supported walking and standing in a therapeutic setting for non-ambulatory children with CP seem to improve participation in activities of daily living and social roles, as well as pulmonary and gastrointestinal functions [22].
3. Improved bone mineral density [23].
4. Less musculoskeletal pain.
5. Reduced risk of hip displacement [9, 10].
6. Lesser risk of pressure sores, aspiration and early death.

2. Goals of treatment

The goals of treatment for persons with severe CP are different from those for ambulatory persons with CP. Persons with severe CP are at increased risk of developing displacement of the hip, spinal deformities and joint contracture, which may altogether hinder and interfere with caregiving, positioning, sitting and transferring the person. Other comorbidities include cognitive disorders, visual and hearing impairment, epilepsy, difficulties in chewing and swallowing, drooling, speech, digestive disorder, respiratory illness and bowel and bladder problems [24].

The management aims [24, 25] of severe CP are to

1. Relieve or prevent pain and discomfort.
2. Facilitate ease of care: dressing, toileting, bathing/hygiene; positioning: seating and lying down; transfers and mobility.
3. Preserve or improve health.
4. Improve the quality of life.

More specific therapeutic goals [26] include the following:

1. Adequate tone control.
2. Straight spine and level pelvis (to allow comfortable sitting and positioning).
3. Stable, enlocated, mobile and painless hips.
4. Mobile knees that can flex to sit and extend to brace for transfer.
5. Plantigrade feet.

3. Treatment options

Management aims of severe CP are very challenging and the ultimate goal of the rehabilitation process is to make the child independent at community and household level. The primary aim is to prevent any secondary complications. The rehabilitation of severe CP is an intensive process in which the patient's goals are prioritised with the help of a team of physiotherapists, occupational therapists, speech therapists, psychologists, special educators, etc., headed by a rehabilitation physician to improve the person's function physically, mentally and socially. This process also requires active participation by the patient and caregivers. No two persons with severe CP are the same. However, the impact of rehabilitation techniques on one person must be taken for reference while rehabilitating the other.

The usual management of severe CP at present consists of physical therapy, sometimes followed by multiple, and often concurrent, medical and surgical interventions, most intensively in early childhood through pre-adolescence. While a growing list of treatments, e.g. oral antispasticity medication, alcohol, phenol or botulinum toxin injections, have been shown to individually improve some motor outcomes, few definitive practice guidelines have been proposed for the management of CP due to limited and fragmented scientific evidence to support multidisciplinary intervention approaches [27]. Persons with severe CP usually do not fulfil the selection criteria for selective dorsal rhizotomy. Intrathecal baclofen is a therapeutic option in this population, but the disadvantages include high cost and serious complications like infection, neurological injury and hip dislocation.

In ambulatory patients (GMFCS levels I, II and III), single-event multilevel surgery (SEMLS) has become widely accepted to be effective in improving gait parameters and the quality of life [28]. However, the effectiveness of orthopaedic surgery (OS) to improve and maintain mobility in children with lower functional levels (GMFCS levels IV and V) has not been ascertained. A study conducted in 2012 revealed that orthopaedic surgery in children with CP at GMFCS IV was unlikely to restore or maintain mobility. The study reported that the following results:

- Only 36.4% of the patients achieved their goals.
- The Functional Mobility Scale (FMS) remained the same in 95.4% of the patients.
- Most children lost their ability to perform assisted walking and standing transfers at 2 years' post-surgery.

The authors concluded that the role of orthopaedic surgery for children with CP at GMFCS level IV is limited to the treatment and prevention of spastic hip disease and scoliosis [29].

The aims of OS in GMFCS level IV are to optimise

1. Foot positioning for standing and walking/transferring.
2. Knee extension for standing and walking/transferring.
3. Hips to prevent progressive sub-luxation and dislocation.

The aims of OS in GMFCS level V are to optimise

1. Foot positioning for feet on footplate of wheelchair.
2. Hips to prevent progressive sub-luxation and dislocation.
3. Other surgery may be indicated if impacting on the persons' quality of life (e.g. pain) or ability to be positioned comfortably in their wheelchair.

None of the conventional therapeutic approaches reported so far have shown any significant improvement in gross motor function or the ability to ambulate in persons with severe CP. Consequently, the recommended rehabilitation strategy across the world at present for severe CP is wheelchair-aided mobility. Hence, there is a strong need to evaluate alternative methods of treatment that can allow assisted ambulation in persons with severe CP.

4. Orthopaedic selective spasticity-control surgery (OSSCS)

OSSCS, a Japanese OS approach, has been proposed with the aims of selective reduction of a specific muscle's spasticity, dystonia and athetosis, and improvement of anti-gravity posture control and movement [30]. The principles of OSSCS are as follows:

1. Longer muscles are selected for surgical release on the assumption that spasticity of shorter muscles limits anti-gravity function in persons with CP.
2. Longer muscles that are considered are always multi-articular and inserted at the more distal portion in the same muscle group.
3. The longer and hyperactive muscle fibres can be selectively sectioned with intramuscular tendon lengthening and controlled sliding tendon lengthening.
4. Simultaneous release of flexor and extensor muscle groups is performed in each joint (except at wrists, hands and feet).

The main surgical techniques in OSSCS are intramuscular release and controlled sliding lengthening [30].

The advantages of OSSCS over conventional OS [30, 31] are as follows:

1. There is no loss of anti-gravity activity and weakness of the muscles because monoarticular muscles are preserved.

2. Over lengthening of tendons is avoided because of the surgical technique of controlled sliding tendon lengthening.
3. It controls spasticity, produces reciprocal movements to facilitate anti-gravity muscles and improves functional skills and voluntary movement of the hand.
4. It leads to significant functional improvement in the severely involved spastic quadriplegia, athetoid or dystonia.
5. There is no loss of sensation or sense of stereognosis.
6. There is no increase in the occurrence of dislocations.

5. Single Event Multilevel Lever Arm Restoration and Anti-Spasticity Surgery (SEMLARASS)

SEMLARASS is an advancement of the concept of OSSCS [32]. The additional principles of SEMLARASS include the following:

1. Operating between the ages of 4 and 6 years (preferably) to avoid joint decompensation and over lengthening of tendons that happen due to continued usage of deformed joints.
2. Simultaneous restoration of lever arm dysfunction (LAD) is essential for spasticity and contracture correction as well as to reduce chances of recurrence of deformities and repeat surgery at a later stage, and to improve the direction of pull of muscles and facilitating strengthening.
3. Minimally invasive procedures using image intensification that do not require large skin incisions and consequent risk of blood loss and infection.
4. Use of only external fixators that do not require a second operation for removal, and are technically superior to internal fixation in enabling reduction of dislocated hips and preventing stress shielding of the bone and consequent fractures after implant removal.
5. All surgeries to restore LAD are extra-articular to allow for the maximum growth potential of children's bones.
6. Power generators are preserved: tendon transfers of spastic muscles may lead to further weakness and worsen, lead to an opposite deformity, e.g. genu recurvatum following Eggers transfer.
7. For non-reducible hip dislocation, the preferred salvage operation is redirection of femoral head and tectoplasty while preserving the femoral head (**Figure 1** and **2**).
8. The surgery is followed by a structured, intensive, institutional, physician-directed, multidisciplinary rehabilitation protocol.

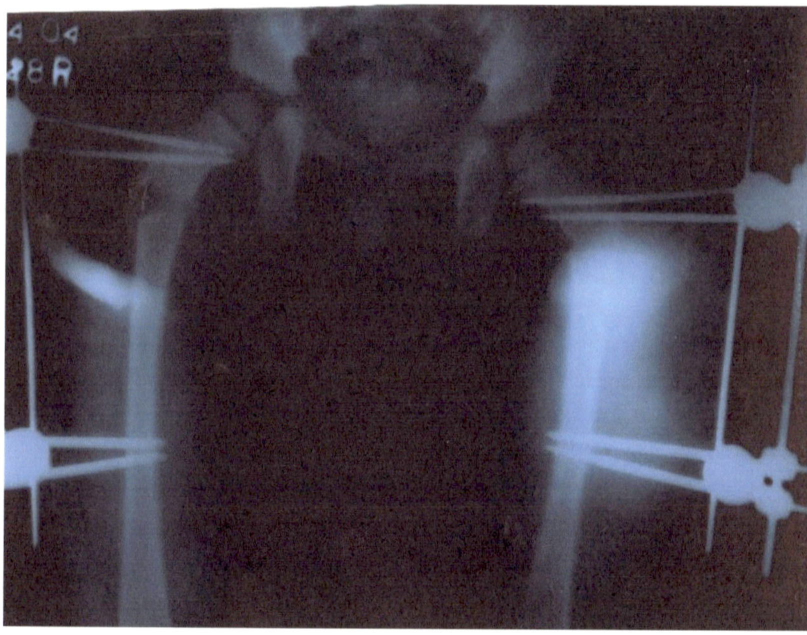

Figure 1. Percutaneous varus derotation osteotomies with external fixators.

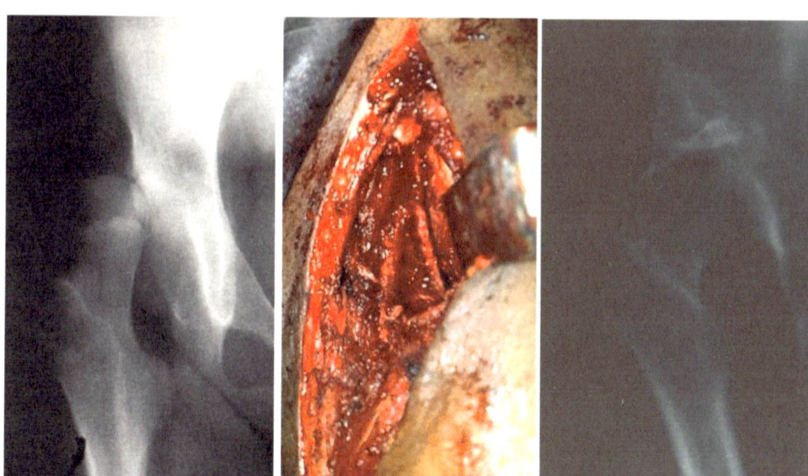

Figure 2. Tectoplasty.

Following are the components of SEMLARASS:

1. Single event: under a single anaesthesia, requiring only one hospital admission and one period of rehabilitation, all surgeries are completed.

2. Multilevel: simultaneous correction of all the affected regions and all orthopaedic deformities (soft tissue and bony) as joints are interdependent.
3. Lever arm restoration: to improve the direction of pull of muscles and to facilitate muscle strengthening post-operatively, LAD corrections are done simultaneously.
4. Anti-spasticity surgery: using the principles of OSSCS.

6. Rehabilitation approaches used with SEMLARASS

SEMLARASS is followed by a protocol-based rehabilitation that has already been published [32]. This rehabilitation approach is comprehensive, and includes physiotherapy, occupational therapy, speech therapy, orthosis and other adaptive equipment, recreational activities, school and education adaptation and psychosocial support, etc. [33]. Rehabilitation in severe CP can differ due to clinical type and severity of conditions, physiological age and socioeconomic factors. In addition, visual, auditory, cognitive disorders, seizures, learning disabilities and emotional problems may influence intervention outcomes [34]. Physiotherapy plays a central role in managing the condition; it focuses on function, movement and optimal use of the person's potential. Physiotherapy uses physical approaches to promote, maintain and restore physical, psychological and social well-being. The rehabilitation occurs not only at the rehabilitation centre but also involves the functional strategies at home, community, school or work and other recreational environments, where the therapists works on making the person with CP to become independent by concentrating on gross motor activities, functional mobility and ambulation either with or without assistive devices [33].

Active rehabilitation has been the choice of functional treatment for CP according to the present evidence available in the literature [35]. The rehabilitation is focussed on a combination of aspects involving physical, mental and social functions. It involves a time-bound interaction between the patient, therapist and other persons involved in the rehabilitation process to show a reduction in the disability on the person's day-to-day activities by his or her condition [36]. Active rehabilitation involves making the person with severe CP active through most of the waking hours and participating actively in the rehabilitation. A variety of therapeutic programmes such as aquatic therapy, virtual reality-based therapy, physiotherapy, occupational therapy, hippotherapy (HT), whole body vibration therapy (WBVT), body-weight-supported treadmill training, EMG biofeedback and functional activity training are used. In addition, supportive therapies such as psychological counselling, special education, neurotherapy, yoga therapy and relaxation exercises also form a part of the treatment regimen. In the post-operative phase, a person with severe CP undergoes 5–6 hours of the above therapies in a programmed manner through a phased multidisciplinary treatment protocol for 6–9 months and less intensively thereafter [32].

6.1. Aquatic therapy

Aquatic therapy is one of the most popular and important rehabilitation strategies in persons with severe CP [37]. Water is an equalising medium; its gravity-minimising nature reduces compressive joint forces, providing a better exercise environment for patients with medical conditions that may restrict physical training on land [38]. Adapted aquatic exercises have been particularly recommended as a part of physical activity programmes for persons with severe CP. The buoyant nature of water provides persons with severe CP the opportunity to feel their bodies free from the constraints they experience on land [39]. Aquatic exercises have benefits on joint range of motion, strength of muscles, pain, muscle spasms, circulation and respiratory function, speech, balance, coordination and posture [40]. Ease of movement and weight relief allows safe movement exploration, strengthening and functional activity training with a reduced level of joint loading and impact, providing a gentler environment for persons who experience persistent abnormal loading [39]. In addition, aquatic physical activities are important for the teaching-learning process and might promote greater independence, better manual ability and, as a consequence, increase social participation in persons with severe CP [41]. Despite the fact that swimming is one of the most frequently reported physical activities in children and adolescents with CP, there is no consensus on optimal concepts of aquatic physical activity regarding duration of intervention period, duration of a single treatment, frequency per week of treatment, individual/group work, water temperature and swimming pool size and depth [38]. In our practice, the aquatic therapy consisted of 5 minutes of light warm-up in the temperature-controlled swimming pool (forward and backward walking, jumping and other such exercises), 20 minutes of exercise on swimming techniques (prone and back gliding from the wall, prone and back floating and blowing bubbles) and 5 minutes of play (ball games, chasing games, etc.). The therapy was focused and performed individually (**Figure 3**). To ensure active participation, the intervention was customised to maximise enjoyment by each individual. Depending on the improved performance demonstrated by each person and related functional ability, the complexity of the exercises was increased. In addition, some interventions focused more on arm movements than on leg movements and vice versa. Thus, the goals and progression of each person could be followed individually, and every instructor was able to easily continue onto the next lesson with each child.

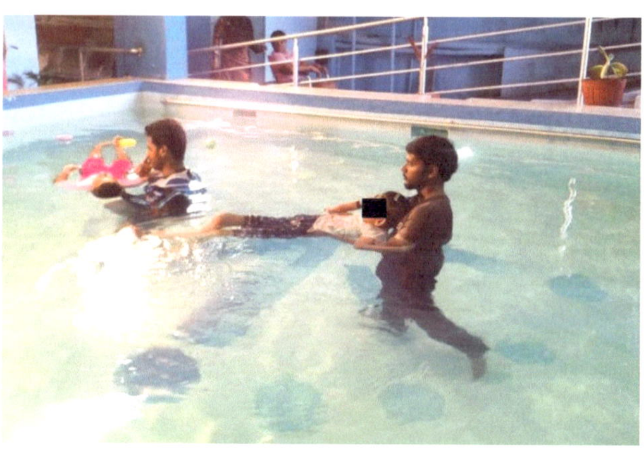

Figure 3. Aquatic therapy.

6.2. Body-weight-supported treadmill training (BWSTT)

Persons with severe CP are non-ambulatory. Treadmill training has shown positive outcomes in improving ambulation in CP [42]. Animal studies of supported treadmill training have demonstrated restoration of coordinated stepping movements in spinalised cats [43]. BWSTT is an active, repetitive, task-specific approach used to facilitate attainment of stepping and locomotion and to achieve a more normalised gait pattern. It is a method of task-oriented ambulatory training using the overhead suspension system and harness to support a percentage of the person's body weight while walking on a treadmill. Other effects of BWSTT include increase in walking speed, improved balance and increased endurance [44]. We use an indigenously constructed BWSTT device to aid persons with severe CP during the gait training phase of rehabilitation (**Figure 4**). The body weight support device can facilitate walking, both on treadmill and on level ground. In addition to its effectiveness in improving the person's walking ability, it also reduces the physical workload of physiotherapists and caregivers handling the persons with severe CP.

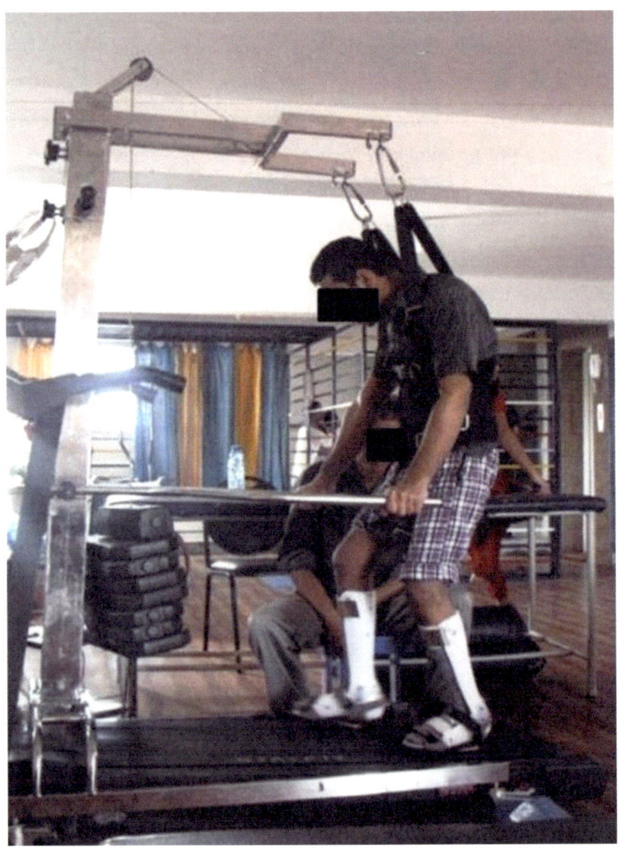

Figure 4. Body-weight-supported treadmill training.

http://dx.doi.org/10.5772/64642

6.3. Functional electrical stimulation (FES)

FES is used to stimulate targeted muscles during ambulation, especially in enhancing quadriceps function, allowing for better range in knee extension. It is used to improve gait control and trunk control [45–47]. Persons with severe CP have difficulty in generating sufficient muscle force. So, combining exercise with FES programme is a good option for increasing the intensity and effectiveness of the strengthening programme. Studies show participants in an FES programme can make measurable gains in body structure and function, activity and participation. The evidence supporting the efficacy of FES in improving gait quality, gait symmetry and muscle strength and motor control in persons with CP is growing steadily [48–51]. Given the complex nature of the gait deviations seen in children with CP, many paediatric FES studies investigate the effect of multi-channel FES systems on abnormal gait. Most multi-channel systems include stimulation of the anterior tibialis muscle as a treatment for drop foot [45, 51, 52]. Two of the FES review studies investigated single-channel FES systems that operate as neuroprostheses by stimulating the peroneal nerve to alleviate drop foot [45, 48]. In our setting also, we use a single-channel FES to facilitate the activation of tibialis anterior and knee extension for gait training, especially during treadmill training (**Figure 5**).

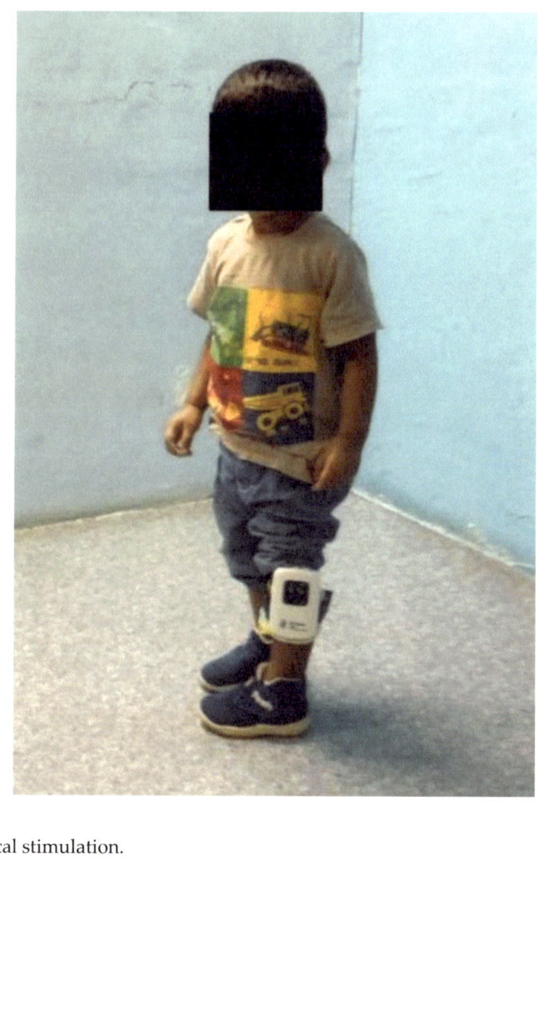

Figure 5. Functional electrical stimulation.

6.4. Whole body vibration therapy (WBVT)

Studies on vibration therapy at a specific frequency and amplitude have many negative effects on humans. However, recent studies have shown that vibration therapy for humans at very low amplitude and frequency is safe and beneficial to the human musculoskeletal structures. WBVT can be used as a form of exercise targeted for improving muscle strength, power, flexibility and coordination. Persons using this tool stand on the vibrating platform so that the whole body was stimulated with a sinusoidal vibration [52]. WBVT has been utilised to deliver mechanical accelerations to the appendicular and axial skeletons to elicit increased bone mass. WBVT has been shown to be specifically effective in improving bone mineral density especially in hip and spine for persons with severe CP after plaster immobilisation [53, 54]. The advantage of WBVT lies in its ability to be applied in a low-impact manner, which is critical for persons with impaired mobility and muscle strength (**Figure 6**). In our practice, WBVT is used, initially with suspension similar to BWSTT, in persons with severe CP who are in the weight bearing phase of rehabilitation.

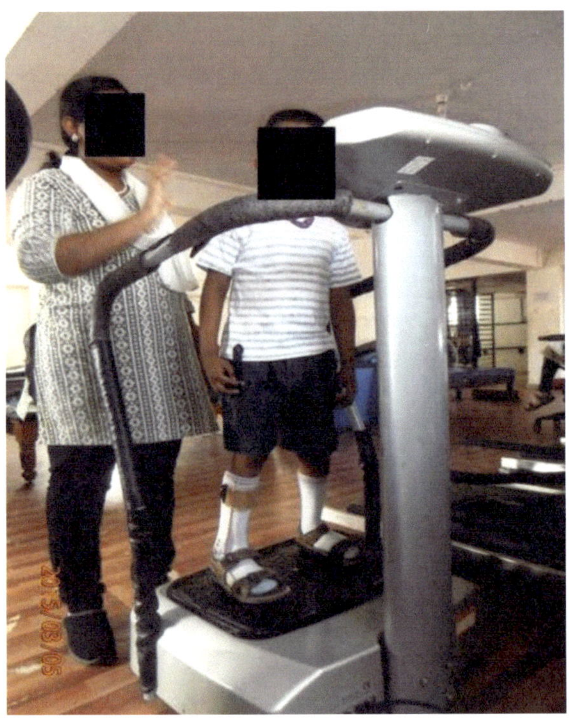

Figure 6. Whole body vibration therapy.

6.5. Virtual reality-based therapy (VRBT)

Virtual reality is the use of interactive simulations using computer hardware and software to present users with opportunities to perform rehabilitation in virtual environments that appear, sound, and less frequently, feel similar to real-world objects and events. The advantage of VRBT is that it allows a more elaborate and complex interaction between the virtual environment and the user. We have reported on the successful use of Nintendo Wii for VRBT to improve the balance, motivation and participation of children with CP following SEMLARASS [55] (**Figure 7**). Virtual reality-based bilateral arm training shows improvement in upper limb motor skills on the affected sites and in bilateral coordination ability. It can also improve trunk control and concentration [56]. Active participation, receiving feedback and repetition of movements during the VRBT intervention, assists in motor learning that induces cortical reorganisation and neural plasticity changes in the brain [57–59]. VRBT also increases the exercise compliance level in achieving selective motor control and enhances the effectiveness of conventional physiotherapy [60]. Participants were highly motivated by the feedback, challenge, variability and other competitive factors involved in the VRBT and overall give a sense of achievement mimicking the real world [61–63]. We also use Microsoft X-Box with Kinect and virtual reality headsets in neurorehabilitation. Initially, suspension is used for non-ambulatory persons.

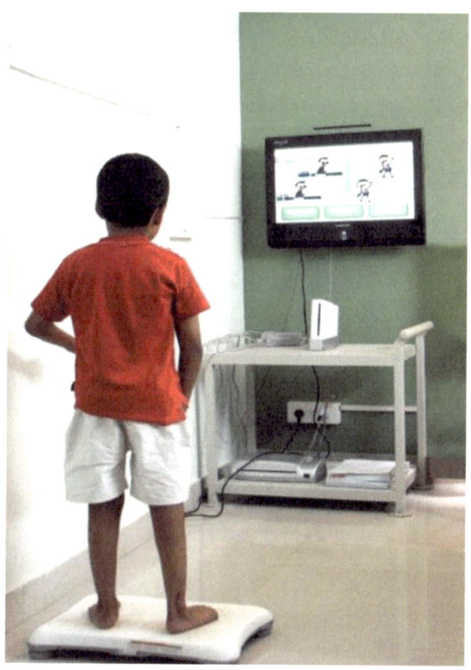

Figure 7. Virtual reality-based therapy.

6.6. EMG biofeedback

Biofeedback uses the principle of measuring and processing normal and/or abnormal neuromuscular activity in the form of auditory or visual feedback by means of an electromechanical instrument. EMG biofeedback specifically uses surface electrodes and records the muscular activity and gives the feedback that can be therapeutically used to facilitate or inhibit the muscular activity. This helps to create a better awareness about the physiological process of the abnormal body movements in specific activities of the individuals. Pressure, temperature, angular and positional systems can also be used as other modes of biofeedback similar to EMG biofeedback [64–67]. EMG biofeedback is now widely used in the rehabilitation of upper motor neuron lesions and also found that it helps in improving the spastic muscles by relaxing them [68–70]. In CP rehabilitation, EMG biofeedback has not been evaluated with any major controlled studies. Studies with small sample sizes have reported reduction in spasticity in the gastrocnemius [71] and increases in active range of motion and ankle dorsiflexion strength [72]. Although EMG is used to reduce muscle spasticity, there was no degree of changes in muscle contracture using EMG biofeedback. However, reversing muscle contracture can be achieved by combining surgical procedures that lengthen the muscles along with biofeedback training in order to maintain the lengthened muscle. [73]. In our setup, we use a single-channel EMG biofeedback device that provides an individual with supplemental information about the response of muscular activity, allowing the individual to attempt to control a given output associated with this process (**Figure 8**). Through trial and error, the person receives feedback on his or her success in adapting their behaviour to achieve the desired output (reduced spasticity or improved muscle strength). A variety of instruments are being used in research and in the clinical setting including surface EMG, computer-assisted feedback and a variety of simple auditory and visual feedback such as providing an auditory cue on the heel of a child to encourage heel-toe gait [74].

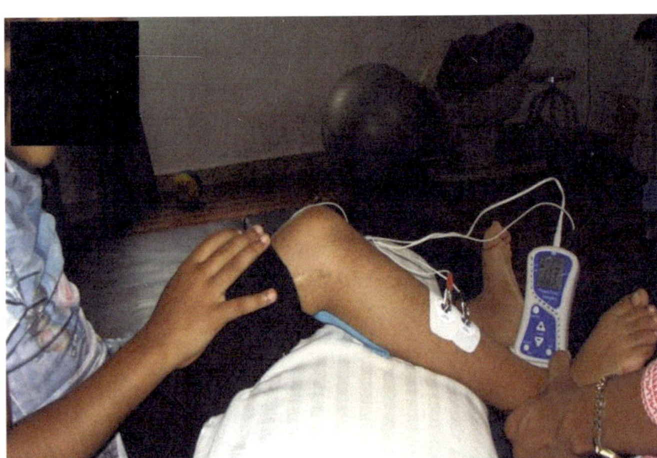

Figure 8. EMG biofeedback.

6.7. Activity monitor (AM)

AMs can be used for persons with severe CP as a biofeedback device, especially in rehabilitation for improving specific gait parameters. It is economical, easy to use and provides a real-

http://dx.doi.org/10.5772/64642

time feedback [75]. Physical activity seems to be one of the most important factors in effective CP rehabilitation or prevention of functional decline in older persons [76]. Small, lightweight, body-worn accelerometers that are able to record activity over longer periods of time now are available commercially. Body positions, movement and number of steps taken by the subject are detected in the sensory systems by inbuilt pre-installed software. This pre-installed software helps to extract data of the body's movement such as no of steps taken, time, speed, kilometers travelled and calories burnt. In our setup, we use a small, lightweight AM worn on persons' body for a particular period of time and subsequently monitoring the output and fixing targets to achieve, thus acting as a biofeedback device for persons with severe CP (**Figure 9**). This accurate measurement of free-living physical activity using advanced dynamic acceleration and inclination logging technology allows medical and rehabilitation professionals to assess patient compliance with exercise and treatment protocols, and also patient response to novel treatment interventions.

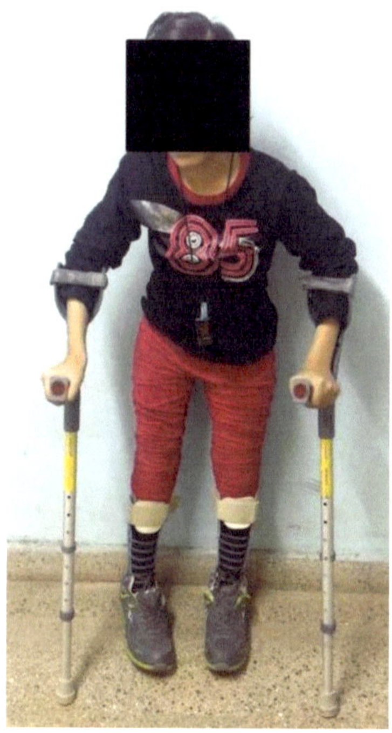

Figure 9. Tracking the training with activity monitor.

6.8. Hippotherapy

HT is a form of physical, occupational or speech therapy utilising a trained horse. The movement of the horse affects a rider's posture, balance, coordination, strength and sensorimotor systems. Recently, mechanical HT devices have been used in the rehabilitation of persons with severe CP. The mechanical HT is the modern form of providing therapeutic horse riding benefits by a pre-programmed mechanically operated device, mimicking a horse riding experience (**Figure 10**). We use mechanical HT to improve head and trunk control, sitting balance, posture and promote functional activities [77–80]. HT should be avoided in the presence of hip displacement or hip osteotomies (till the stage of bony consolidation).

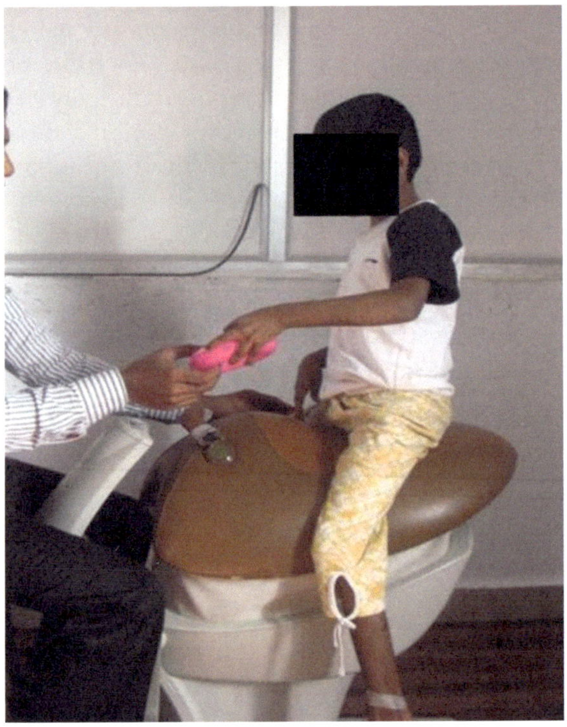

Figure 10. Mechanical Hippotherapy.

6.9. Velcro platform (VP)

Persons with CP often have difficulty in balancing post-SEMLARASS. VP is a novel method developed and designed by us for improving standing balance. The principle behind the use of Velcro for increasing the stability of base of support was that the sensory input from the varied rehabilitation strategies using Velcro for support helps in increased muscular activation, thereby improving functional performance [81]. The majority of persons with severe CP have severe muscular weakness and fear of falling, post-SEMLARASS, and have difficulties in achieving standing balance. VP consists of a wide wooden board attached with foot-contoured pads enforced with straps that accommodate the person's feet. The positive and negative pieces of a conventional Velcro form the contact surfaces of the platform base and the foot pads. The person is made to stand on the board fastening the Velcro straps. The device provides better foot contact to the ground, which aids in better weight bearing, proper biomechanical alignment and acts as an indirect psychological assistance, which can make a person stand independently without or with minimal manual assistance (**Figure 11**). It helps to reduce the gravitational insecurities, fear of falling and gives confidence to a patient. Although the pilot study reported significant improvement in balance parameters and reduction in fear of falls, a larger clinical trial investigating the effectiveness of the VP is under progress.

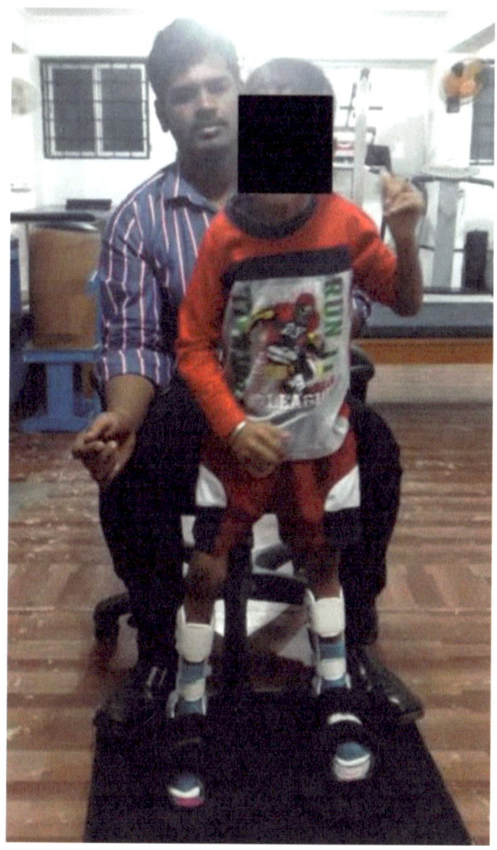

Figure 11. Balance training with Velcro platform.

6.10. Head-held laser illumination device (HHLID)

Similar to VP, HHLID is also an indigenously developed device that can be a useful tool in the post-SEMLARASS rehabilitation programme for the improvement of sitting or standing balance and head or trunk control in persons with severe CP. A Laser-pointer-based focussed trajectory exercises were found to improve the hip extensor activation in comparison to erector spinae activation during pelvic bridging exercise [82]. A laser pointer device attached to the pelvis has been used to assess impaired balance [83]. HHLID consists of a laser-emitting device that can be fixed to the person's head or pelvis and the target is to focus on a variable screen with mazes that challenges the person's balance and control abilities (**Figure 12**). HHLID works by giving visual feedback and it requires active correction of the patient, initially guided and assisted by the physiotherapist. The pilot study reported significant improvements in sitting balance, and a larger clinical trial investigating the effectiveness of the HHLID is under progress.

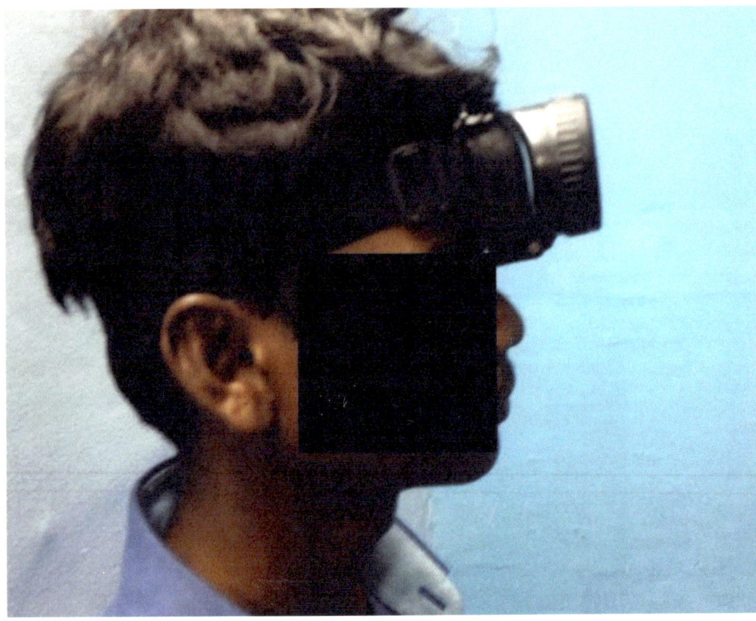

Figure 12. Child fixed with a head held laser illumination device.

6.11. Gaze-assistive rehabilitation technology (GART)

Gaze stabilisation during head motion is an important aspect of rehabilitation of individuals with severe physical impairments with problems in communication and speech disorders. For such persons, gaze stabilisation and control-based technological devices help in communication and interaction without the use of upper or lower extremities [84]. GART works on the principle of video-based corneal reflection eye trackers [85]. A few studies have reported the use of GART in severe CP helping them perform certain activities and increase participation [86, 87]. We are currently studying the Samsung EyeCan+ eye mouse, a futuristic device that enables people with severe CP to use computers only through eye movements. The EyeCan+ is a simple portable box positioned near the computer monitor and users are not required to wear glasses or other special equipment. Users can work with the device either sitting or lying down and just need to be a couple of feet from the monitor. This device allows people to compose and edit documents as well as browse the web (click, double click, scroll, drag, etc.) through simple eye movements. Eighteen different mouse menus allow the person with severe CP to communicate, play games and participate in rehabilitation (**Figure 13**).

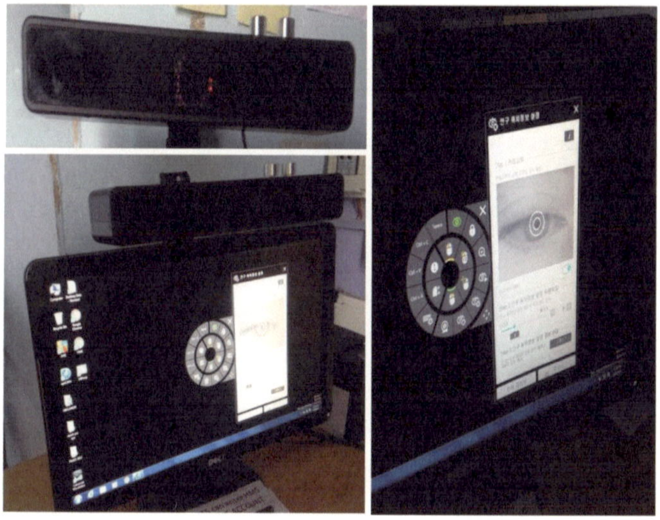

Figure 13. EyeCan+ device fixed to a personal computer.

Other supportive therapies in the rehabilitation protocol include occupational therapy involving specific goal-oriented therapies such as constraint-induced movement therapy (CIMT), mirror therapy, play therapy, music and art therapy, psychological counselling, behavioural training, special education, yoga therapy, speech therapy and dance movement therapy.

6.12. Results of SEMLARASS for severe CP

A study was conducted on 170 children with severe CP (GMFCS levels IV and V) to find out the functional outcome of SEMLARASS and rehabilitation. The mean age of the participants was 9.68 ± 4.77 years. The follow-up ranged from 2 to 10 years (mean = 4 years). The outcome measures such as component of Gross Motor Function Measure (GMFM-88), Functional Mobility Scale, Physicians Rating Scale (PRS), Manual Ability Classification System (MACS) were used to compare the functional status of the child before and after SEMLARASS.

The results showed a significant improvement in all GMFM-88 components and the values were lying and rolling (A): GMFM 5: t-9.77 ($P < 0.001$); GMFM 4: t-8.56 ($P < 0.001$); sitting (B): GMFM 5: t-20.01 ($P < 0.001$); GMFM 4: t-12.61 ($P < 0.001$); crawling and kneeling (C): GMFM 5: t-22.26 ($P < 0.001$); GMFM 4: t-21.01 ($P < 0.001$); standing (D): GMFM 5: t-20.01 ($P < 0.001$); GMFM 4: t-22.64 ($P < 0.001$); standing (D): GMFM 5: t-20.01 ($P < 0.001$); GMFM 4: t-22.64 ($P < 0.001$); walking, running and jumping (E): GMFM 5: t-12.71 ($P < 0.001$); GMFM 4: t-15.65 ($P < 0.001$) and total GMFM-88: GMFM 5: t-31.55 ($P < 0.001$); GMFM 4: t-32.86 ($P < 0.001$), respectively. The result of pre-post PRS evaluation showed a significant improvement for both sides ($P < 0.01$). Correlation studies showed median value of Functional Mobility Scale of 1 before surgery and 3 after surgery. Before surgery the median value of Gross Motor Functional Classification System was level IV and after surgery it was level II. The GMFCS improved two levels on average. Before surgery, the mean value of Pediatric QOL (PQOL) was 23.11 ± 14.02; after surgery, the mean value was 39.64 ± 17.49. Before surgery median value of Manual Ability Classification System was 3 and after surgery it was 1. No child was wheelchair bound at the end of the rehabilitation and all the children were able to walk at least with help of a walking aid. A significant improvement was noted in their participation levels, motivation and a significant improvement in the overall quality of life [88]. Over 50 patients have been followed up for 10 years and there have been no significant recurrence of deformities or significant deterioration of gross motor function.

7. Discussion

The currently practised treatment options have little impact on gross motor function and mobility in non-ambulatory persons with spastic quadriplegia and dyskinetic CP, which constitute nearly 70% of all cases of CP. In particular, OS is considered to have minimal role in this patient population. A retrospective cohort study of 107 children with bilateral spastic CP, classified as GMFCS level II or III, who underwent surgery at a single tertiary institution in Australia between 1997 and 2008, reported that the GMFCS levels remained stable and unchanged in 95% of children and improved by one level in 5% of children [89]. Khan reported a series of previously untreated 85 non-walker children with diplegic CP who underwent multilevel surgery. All patients improved and became walkers. However, since the GMFCS was not used, their cohort cannot be compared to this study [90]. Blumetti et al. found a low rate of success after surgery in patients with GMFCS level IV with only 36.4% of the patients achieving their goals. The FMS scores remained the same in 95.4% of the patients. Only one patient maintained an FMS score of 2, 1, 1 at 2 years' follow-up. Most children lost their ability to do supported walking and standing transfers at 2 years' post-surgery [29]. Some external factors are known to influence the outcomes after OS, including post-operative rehabilitation, use of orthotic devices, pain-controlling strategies, adequate tone control, and presence of co-morbidities [91]. However, all patients in this series received a standardised rehabilitation programme as described previously and were closely monitored by the team of medical and rehabilitation professionals. Unlike previous studies the current study showed that GMFCS levels improved at least by two levels and significant improvement in gross motor function and mobility was recorded. The main limitation of the study was the lack of a control group.

8. Conclusion

A well-planned and executed SEMLARASS, followed by intensive, protocol-based, sequenced multidisciplinary active rehabilitation, provides the person with severe CP, a significant functional improvement in gross motor function and mobility. SEMLARASS is the only documented treatment for CP till date that has been able to address all the three key problems in CP—selective reduction of spasticity, dyskinetic movements and LAD. The best age for SEMLARASS is 4–6 years before the LAD become severe or joints become decompensated.

http://dx.doi.org/10.5772/64642

Intensive, protocol-based and medically supervised rehabilitation for several years and close follow-up are needed at least till skeletal maturity. SEMLARASS provides a patient with severe CP with the best hope for a dramatic, predictable and lasting functional improvement.

9. Case study 1

9.1. Pre-op status

(A) A 13-year-old girl with spastic quadriplegia was confined to bed and completely dependent on caregivers for all her daily activities. She had no neck control or sitting balance. When held upright by an adult, there was severe crouching at hips and knees. Her GMFCS level was V.

9.2. Treatment

She underwent SEMLARASS in two stages: the first stage with OSCSS of bilateral hamstring, psoas, rectus femoris and gracilis along with femoral derotation and tibial derotation osteotomies and the second stage (after 8 weeks) with OSCSS of bilateral forearm flexors, pronators and hand intrinsics.

9.3. Current functional status

At a follow-up of 13 months, she was able to walk with the assistance of walker with forearm gutter. She was able to sit independently either long or cross sitting and able to perform some of her daily activities such as feeding, brushing and upper body dressing on her own. Her present GMFCS score was III (**Figure 14**).

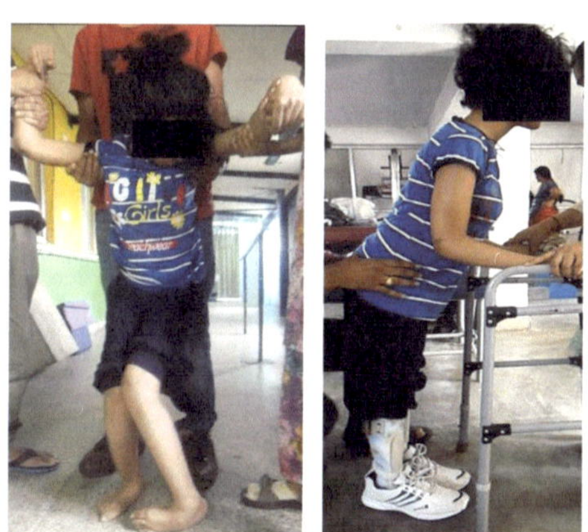

Figure 14. Pre- and post-rehabilitation status of child A.

'Our daughter, till the age of 12, could only sit with maximal support. But after SEMLARASS and intensive rehabilitation in RECOUP, our daughter is now able to sit without support in both cross sitting and long sitting and now she is able to stand and walk with walking frame with minimum support. She now feels more confident'—parents of A.

10. Case study 2

10.1. Pre-op status

(S) A 12-year-old boy with spastic diplegia was not able to walk and perform his daily activities. His GMFCS level was IV.

10.2. Treatment

He underwent SEMLARASS with OSCSS of bilateral hamstring, psoas and rectus femoris along with bilateral femoral varus derotation osteotomy.

10.3. Current functional status

At a follow-up of 12 months, he was able to walk independently for over 100 metres and able to climb up stairs by holding the hand rails and started going to school independently. Current GMFCS score was 2 (**Figure 15**).

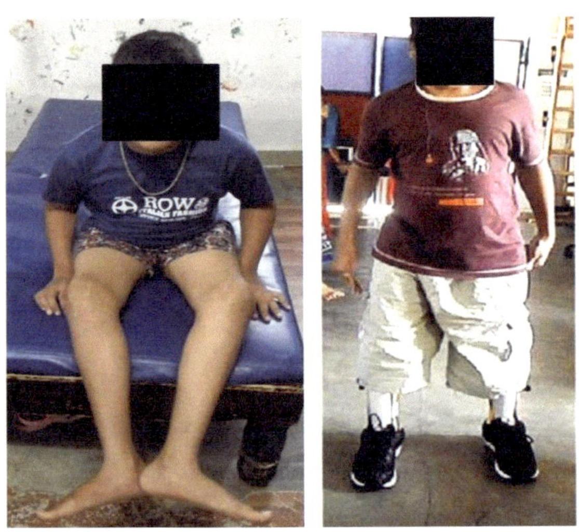

Figure 15. Pre- and post-rehabilitation status of child S.

'Our son, born with Spastic Diplegia, could not walk and needed constant support even for few steps and frequent falls and imbalance were a constant issue. Now, after the treatment at

http://dx.doi.org/10.5772/64642

RECOUP, he started walking independently with lot of confidence and enthusiasm'—parents of S.

11. Case study 3

11.1. Pre-op status

(D) A 6-year-old girl with spastic quadriplegia and bilateral hip dislocations was confined to bed and could only bunny hop or creep from one point to other and was totally dependent on caregivers. Her GMFCS level was IV.

11.2. Treatment

She underwent SEMLARASS in two stages: the first stage with OSCSS of bilateral hamstring, psoas, rectus femoris, gracilis and tibialis anterior along with femoral varus derotation and tibial derotation osteotomies and the second stage (after 8 weeks) with OSCSS of bilateral forearm flexors and pronators.

11.3. Current functional status

After 12 months of follow-up, she was able to walk independently with walker and able to sit up in bed by herself and stand to sit with support. She was able to carry out some basic activities of daily living by her own. Her current GMFCS score was III (**Figure 16**).

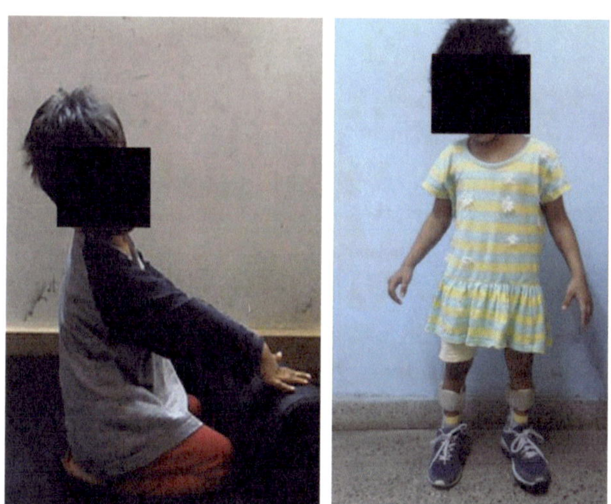

Figure 16. Pre- and post-rehabilitation status of child D.

'The SEMLARASS surgery and rehabilitation at RECOUP had made a lot of difference in her and now she can walk with a walker'—parents of D.

12. Case study 4

12.1. Pre-op status

(MA) A 13-year-old boy with spastic dystonic quadriplegia could not walk, even with support. His GMFCS level was IV.

12.2. Treatment

He underwent SEMLARASS in two stages: the first stage with OSCSS of bilateral hamstring, psoas, rectus femoris and gracilis along with bilateral femoral derotation and tibial derotation osteotomies and the second stage (after 8 weeks) with OSCSS of bilateral forearm flexors and pronators.

12.3. Current functional status

At a follow-up of 10 months, he was able to walk independently using walking frame. He is now able to climb up stairs with 50% assistance. His current GMFCS status was III (**Figure 17**).

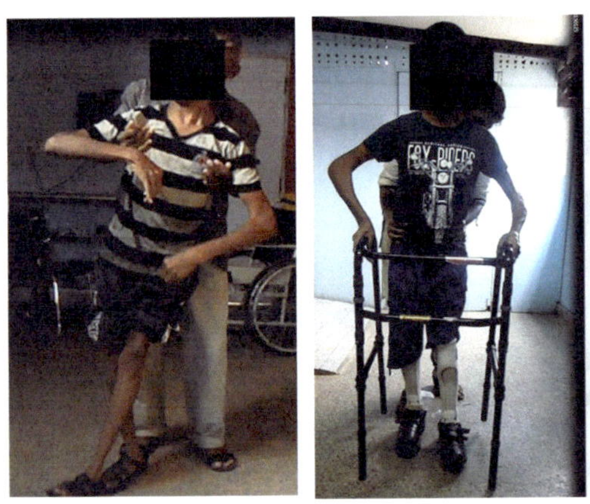

Figure 17. Pre- and post-rehabilitation status of child MA.

'Our son could only walk on toes with his knee bent and used to get a lot of pain and confined to bed. But now, after the surgery and intensive rehabilitation at RECOUP, he started walking independently with a walker and looking for a brighter future ahead'—parents of MA.

13. Case study 5

13.1. Pre-op status

(R) A 5-year-old boy with spastic athetoid quadriplegia with bilateral dislocated hips was not able to sit or stand or use his hands. His GMFCS level was V.

13.2. Treatment

He underwent SEMLARASS with OSCSS of bilateral hamstring, psoas and rectus femoris along with femoral varus derotation osteotomy.

13.3. Current functional status

After 7 years of follow-up, he was able to stand with minimal support and walk with rollator independently. He was now able to climb up stairs with assistance and able to walk on ramp with rollator. His current GMFCS was III (**Figure 18**).

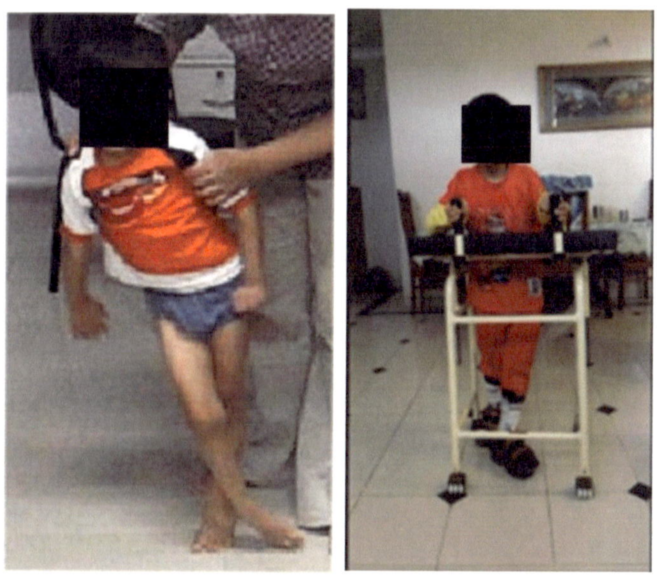

Figure 18. Pre- and post-rehabilitation status of child R.

'Our son born with spastic athetoid quadriplegia till the age of 5 and was not able to sit, stand or walk; after surgery and intensive rehabilitation in RECOUP, our son is now able to sit and stand independently and walk with rollator more confidently'—parents of R.

Author details

Deepak Sharan*, Joshua Samuel Rajkumar, Rajarajeshwari Balakrishnan and Amruta Kulkarni

*Address all correspondence to: deepak.sharan@recoup.in

RECOUP Neuromusculoskeletal Rehabilitation Centre, Bangalore, Karnataka, India

References

[1] Rosenbaum P, Paneth N, Leviton A, Goldstein M, Bax M, Damiano D, Dan B, Jacobsson B. A report: the definition and classification of cerebral palsy. Dev Med Child Neurol. 2007;109(Suppl.):8–14.

[2] Oskoui M, Coutinho F, Dykeman J, Jetté N, Pringsheim T. An update on the prevalence of cerebral palsy: a systematic review and meta-analysis. Dev Med Child Neurol. 2013;55(6):509–519.

[3] Kent R. Chapter 38: Cerebral Palsy. In Barnes MP, Good DC, editors. Handbook of Clinical Neurology. Elsevier. Amsterdam. 2013; pp. 443–459.

[4] Baxter P. Definition and classification of cerebral palsy. Dev Med Child Neurol Suppl.. 2007;49(s2); pp. 8–14.

[5] Palisano RJ, Rosenbaum P, Bartlett D, Livingston MH. Content validity of the expanded and revised gross motor function classification system. Dev Med Child Neurol. 2008;50:744–750.

[6] Singhi PD, Ray M, Suri G. Clinical spectrum of cerebral palsy in north India—an analysis of 1,000 cases. J Trop Pediatr. 2002;48(3):162–166.

[7] Bleck EE. Management of Motor Disorder in Children with Cerebral Palsy. Philadelphia, JB Lippencott, 1984.

[8] Bagg MR, Farber J, Miller F. Long-term follow-up of hip subluxation in cerebral palsy patients. J Pediatr Orthop. 1993;13:32–36.

[9] Hagglund G, Andersson S, Duppe H, Lauge-Pedersen H, Nordmark E, Westbom L. Prevention of dislocation of the hip in children with cerebral palsy: the first ten years of a population-based programme. J Bone Joint Surg. 2005;87B:95–101.

[10] Soo B, Howard JJ, Boyd RN, Reid SM, Lanigan A, Wolfe R, Reddihough D, Graham HK. Hip displacement in cerebral palsy. J Bone Joint Surg Am. 2006;88:121–129.

[11] Hodgkinson I, Jindrich ML, Duhaut P, Vadot JP, Metton G, Berard C. Hip pain in 234 non-ambulatory adolescents and young adults with cerebral palsy: a cross-sectional multicentre study. Dev Med Child Neurol. 2001;43:806–808.

[12] Alriksson-Schmidt A, Hägglund G. Pain in children and adolescents with cerebral palsy—a population based registry study. Acta Paediatr. 2016 Feb 16. doi: 10.1111/apa. 13368. [Epub ahead of print]

[13] King W, Levin R, Schmidt R, Oestreich A, Heubi JE. Prevalence of reduced bone mass in children and adults with spastic quadriplegia. Dev Med Child Neurol. 2003;45:12–16.

[14] Jahnsen R, Villien L, Egeland T, Stanghelle JK, Holm I. Locomotion skills in adults with cerebral palsy. Clin Rehabil. 2004;18:309–316.

[15] Andren E, Grimby G. Dependence in daily activities and life satisfaction in adult subjects with cerebral palsy or spina bifida: a follow-up study. Disabil Rehabil. 2004;26:528–536.

[16] van der Dussen L, Nieuwstraten W, Roebroeck M, Stam HJ. Functional level of young adults with cerebral palsy. Clin Rehabil. 2001;15:84–91.

[17] Michelsen SI, Uldall P, Kejs AM, Madsen M. Education and employment prospects in cerebral palsy. Dev Med Child Neurol. 2005;47:511–517.

[18] Michelsen SI, Uldall P, Hansen T, Madsen M. Social integration of adults with cerebral palsy. Dev Med Child Neurol. 2006;48:643–649.

[19] Schenker R, Coster W, Parush S. Participation and activity performance of students with cerebral palsy within the school environment. Disabil Rehabil. 2005;27:539–552.

[20] Donkervoort M, Roebroeck M, Wiegerink D, van der Heijden-Maessen H, Stam H. Determinants of functioning of adolescents and young adults with cerebral palsy. Disabil Rehabil. 2007;29:453–463.

[21] Sharan D, Ajeesh PS, Rameshkumar R, Manjula M. Musculoskeletal disorders in caregivers of children with cerebral palsy following a multilevel surgery. Work. 2012;41(Suppl. 1):1891–1895.

[22] Eisenberg S, Zuk L, Carmeli E, Katz-Leurer M. Contribution of stepping while standing to function and secondary conditions among children with cerebral palsy. Pediatr Phys Ther. 2009;21(1):79–85.

[23] Hough JP, Boyd RN, Keating JL. Systematic review of interventions for low bone mineral density in children with cerebral palsy. Pediatrics. 2010;125(3):e670–e678.

[24] Narayanan UG, Fehlings D, Weir S, Knights S, Kiran S, Campbell K. Initial development and validation of the caregiver priorities and child health index of life with disabilities (CPCHILD). Dev Med Child Neurol. 2006;48(10):804–812.

[25] Narayanan UG. Lower limb deformity in neuromuscular disorders: pathophysiology, assessment, goals, and principles of management. In Sabharwal S, editors. Pediatric Lower Limb Deformities: Principles and Techniques of Management. Switzerland, Springer. 1st ed., 2016; pp. 267–296.

[26] Gage JR, Novacheck TF. An update on the treatment of gait problems in cerebral palsy. J Pediatric Orthop. 2001;10(4):265–274.

[27] Damiano Dl, Alter KE, Chambers H. New clinical and research trends in lower extremity management for ambulatory children with cerebral palsy. Phys Med Rehabil Clin N Am. 2009;20(3):469–491.

[28] Thompson P, Baker R, Dodd K, Taylor N, Selber P, Wolfe R, Graham HK. Single event multilevel surgery in children with spastic diplegia: a pilot randomized. J Bone Joint Surg Am. 2001;93(5):451–460

[29] Blumetti FC, Wu JCN, Bau KV, Martin B, Hobson SA, Axt MW, Selber P. Orthopedic surgery and mobility goals for children with cerebral palsy GMFCS level IV: what are we setting out to achieve? J Child Orthop. 2012, 6:485–490.

[30] Matsuo T. Cerebral Palsy: Spasticity-Control and Orthopaedics—An Introduction to Orthopaedic Selective Spasticity-Control Surgery (OSSCS). Tokyo: Soufusha; 2002.

[31] Kondo I, Hosokawa K, Iwata M, Oda A, Nomura T, Ikeda K, et al. Effectiveness of selective muscle release surgery for children with cerebral palsy: longitudinal and stratified analysis. Dev Med Child Neurol. 2004;46:540–547.

[32] Sharan D. Neuromusculoskeletal Rehabilitation of Cerebral Palsy Using SEMLARASS. In Emira Svraka, editors. Cerebral Palsy—Challenges for the Future. Rijeka, Croatia, Intech. 2014, Chapter 6; pp. 193–215.

[33] Anttila H, Autti-Rämö I, Suoranta J, Mäkelä M, Malmivaara A. Effectiveness of physical therapy interventions for children with cerebral palsy: a systematic review. BMC Pediatr. 2008;24(8):14.

[34] Butler C, Chambers H, Goldstein M, Harris S, Leach J, Campbell S, Adams R, Darrah J. Evaluating research in developmental disabilities: a conceptual framework for reviewing treatment outcomes. Dev Med Child Neurol. 1999;41(1):55–59.

[35] Novak I, McIntyre S, Morgan C, Campbell L, Dark L, Morton N, Stumbles E, Wilson SA, Goldsmith S. A systematic review of interventions for children with cerebral palsy: state of the evidence. Dev Med Child Neurol. 2013;55(10):885–910.

[36] Royal College of Physicians. Medical Rehabilitation in 2011 and Beyond. Report of a Working Party. RCP, London. 2010. ISBN 978-1-86016-386-9.

[37] Getz M, Hutzler Y. Vermeer A. The effects of aquatic intervention on perceived physical competence and social acceptance in children with cerebral palsy. Eur J Spec Need Educ. 2007;22 (2):217–228.

[38] Gerter JW, Currie SJ. Aquatic exercise programs for children and adolescents with cerebral palsy: what we do know and where do we go? Int J Ped. 2011;2011:712165.

[39] Kelly M, Darrah J. Aquatic exercise for children with cerebral palsy. Dev Med Child Neurol. 2005;47(12):838–842.

[40] Fragala-Pinkham M, Haley SM, O'Neil ME. Group aquatic aerobic exercise for children with disabilities. Dev Med Child Neurol. 2008;50(11):822–827.

[41] Aidar FJ, Silva AJ, Reis VM, Carneiro AL, Vianna JM, Novaes GS. Aquatic activities for severe cerebral palsy people and relation with the teach-learning process. Fit Perf J. 2007;6(6):377–381.

[42] LePage C, Noreau L, Bernard PM. Association between characteristics of locomotion and accomplishment of life habits in children with cerebral palsy. Phys Ther. 1989;78:458–469.

[43] Lovely RG, Gregor RJ, Roy RR, Edgerton VR. Effects of training on the recovery of full weight-bearing stepping in the adult spinal cat. Exp Neurol. 1986;92:421–435.

[44] Mutlu A, Krosschell K, GaeblerSpira D. Treadmill training with partial body-weight support in children with cerebral palsy: a systematic review. Dev Med Child Neurol. 2009;51:268–275.

[45] Khamis S,Martikaro R,Wientroub S,Hemo Y,Hayek S. A functional electrical stimulation system improves knee control in crouch gait. J Child Orthop. 2015;9(2):137–143.

[46] Postans NJ,Granat MH. Effect of functional electrical stimulation, applied during walking, on gait in spastic cerebral palsy. Dev Med Child Neurol. 2005;47:46–52.

[47] Karabay İ,Dogan A,Arslan MD,Dost G,Ozgirgin N. Effects of functional electrical stimulation on trunk control in children with diplegic cerebral palsy. Disabil Rehabil. 2012;34(11):965–970.

[48] Johnston TE, Finson RL, McCarthy JJ, Smith BT, Betz RR, Mulcahey MJ. Use of functional electrical stimulation to augment traditional orthopaedic surgery in children with cerebral palsy. J Pediatr Orthop. 2004;24:283–291.

[49] Karabay I, Oztürk GT, Malas FU, Kara M, Tiftik T, Ersöz M, Ozçakar L. Short-term effects of neuromuscular electrical stimulation on muscle architecture of the tibialis anterior and gastrocnemius in children with cerebral palsy: preliminary results of a prospective controlled study. Am J Phys Med Rehabil. 2015;94(9):728–733.

[50] Orlin MN, Pierce SR, Laughton Stackhouse C, Smith BT, Johnston TE, Shewokis PA, McCarthy JJ. Immediate effect of percutaneous intramuscular stimulation during gait in children with cerebral palsy: a feasibility study. Dev Med Child Neurol. 2005;47:684–690.

[51] Pierce SR, Laughton CA, Smith BT, Orlin MN, Johnston TE, McCarthy JJ. Direct effect of percutaneous electric stimulation during gait in children with hemiplegic cerebral palsy: a report of 2 cases. Arch Phys Med Rehabil. 2004;85:339–343.

[52] Seifart A, Unger M, Burger M. Functional electrical stimulation to lower limb muscles after Botox in children with cerebral palsy. Pediatr Phys Ther. 2010;22:199–206.

[53] Ho CL, Holt KG, Saltzman E, Wagenaar RC. Functional electrical stimulation changes dynamic resources in children with spastic cerebral palsy. Phys Ther. 2006;86:987–1000.

[54] Prisby RD, Lafage-Proust MH, Malaval L, Belli A, Vico L. Effects of whole body vibration on the skeleton and other organ systems in man and animal models: what we know and what we need to know. Ageing Res Rev. 2008;7(4):319–329.

[55] Rubin C, Pope M, Fritton JC, Magnusson M, Hansson T, McLeod K. Transmissibility of 15-Hertz to 35-Hertz vibrations to the human hip and lumbar spine: determining the

physiologic feasibility of delivering low-level anabolic mechanical stimuli to skeletal regions at greatest risk of fracture because of osteoporosis. Spine. 2003;28(23):2621–2627.

[56] Semler O, Fricke O, Vezyroglou K, Stark C, Schoenau E. Preliminary results on the mobility after whole body vibration in immobilized children and adolescents. J Musculoskelet Neuronal Interact. 2007;7(1):77–81.

[57] Sharan D, Ajeesh PS, Rameshkumar R, Mathankumar M, Paulina RJ, Manjula M. Virtual reality based therapy for post operative rehabilitation of children with cerebral palsy. Work. 2012;41:3612–3615.

[58] Do JH,Yoo EY, Jung MY, Park HY. The effects of virtual reality based bilateral arm training on hemiplegic children's upper limb motor skills. Neuro Rehabil. 2016;38(2):115–127.

[59] Riener, R. and M. Harders. Virtual Reality for Rehabilitation. In Virtual Reality in Medicine. Springer. London. 2012; pp. 161–180.

[60] You SH, Jang SH, Kim YH, Kwon YH, Barrow I, Hallett M. Cortical reorganization induced by virtual reality therapy in a child with hemiparetic cerebral palsy. Dev Med Child Neurol. 2005;47(9):628–635.

[61] Huang HH, Fetters L, Hale J, McBride A. Bound for success: a systematic review of constraint-induced movement therapy in children with cerebral palsy supports improved arm and hand use. Phys Ther. 2009;89(11):1126–1141.

[62] Bryanton C, Bossé J, Brien M, McLean J, McCormick A, Sveistrup H. Feasibility, motivation, and selective motor control: virtual reality compared to conventional home exercise in children with cerebral palsy. Cyberpsychol Behav. 2006;9(2):123–128.

[63] Harris K, Reid D. The influence of virtual reality play on children's motivation. Can J Occup Ther. 2005;72(1):21–29.

[64] Meyer-Heim A, van Hedel HJ. Robot-assisted and computer-enhanced therapies for children with cerebral palsy: current state and clinical implementation. Semin Pediatr Neurol. 2013;20(2):139–145.

[65] Weiss PL, Bialik P, Kizony R. Virtual reality provides leisure time opportunities for young adults with physical and intellectual disabilities. Cyberpsychol Behav. 2003;6(3):335–342.

[66] Dursun E, Hamamcı N, Donmez S. Angular biofeedback device for sitting balance of stroke patients. Stroke. 1996;27(8):1354–1357.

[67] Ceceli E, Dursun E, Cakci A. Comparison of joint-position biofeedback and conventional therapy methods in genu recurvatum after stroke—6 months' follow-up. Eur J Phys Med Rehabil. 1996;6(5):141–144.

[68] Nichols DS. Balance retraining after stroke using force platform biofeedback. Phys Ther. 1997;77(5):553–558.

[69] Marcus DA, Scharff L, Mercer S, Turk DC. Nonpharmacological treatment for migraine: incremental utility of physical therapy with relaxation and thermal biofeedback. Cephalalgia. 1998;18(5):266–272.

[70] Schleenbaker RE, Mainous III AG. Electromyographic biofeedback for neuromuscular reeducation in the hemiplegic stroke patient: a meta-analysis. Arch Phys Med Rehabil. 1993;74(12):1301–1304.

[71] Wolf SL, Binder-MacLeod SA. Electromyographic biofeedback applications to hemiplegic patient: changes in upper extremity neuromuscular and functional status. Phy Ther. 1983;63:1404–1413.

[72] Moreland JD, Thomson MA, Fuoco AR. Electromyographic biofeedback to improve lower extremity function after stroke: a meta-analysis. Arch Phys Med Rehabil. 1998;79(2):134–140.

[73] Nash J, Neilson PD, O'Dwyer NJ. Reducing spasticity to control muscle contracture of children with cerebral palsy. Dev Med Child Neurol. 1989;31:471–480.

[74] Toner LV, Cook K, Elder GC. Improved ankle function in children with cerebral palsy after computer-assisted motor learning. Dev Med Child Neurol. 1998;40(12):829–835.

[75] O'Dwyer NJ, Neilson PD, Nash J. Reduction of spasticity in cerebral palsy using feedback of the tonic stretch reflex: a controlled study. Dev Med Child Neurol. 1994;36:770–786.

[76] Hartveld A, Hegarty J. Frequent weight shift practice with computerised feedback by cerebral palsied children—four single-case experiments. Physiotherapy 1996;82(10): 573–580.

[77] Mackey AH, Hewart P, Walt SE, Stott NS. The sensitivity and specificity of an activity monitoring detecting functional activities in young people with cerebral palsy. Arch Phys Med Rehabil. 2009;90(8):1396–1401.

[78] Stessman J, Hammerman-Rozenberg R, Cohen A, et al. Physical activity, function, and longevity among the very old. Arch Intern Med. 2009;169:1476–1483.

[79] Kwon JY, Chang HJ, Yi SH, Lee JY, Shin HY, Kim YH. Effect of hippotherapy on gross motor function in children with cerebral palsy: a randomized controlled trial. J Altern Complement Med. 2015;21(1):15–21.

[80] Park ES, Rha DW, Shin JS, Kim S, Jung S. Effects of hippotherapy on gross motor function and functional performance of children with cerebral palsy. Yonsei Med J. 2014;55(6):1736–1742.

[81] Pantall A, Teulier C, Ulrich BD. Changes in muscle activation patterns in response to enhanced sensory input during treadmill stepping in infants born with myelomeningocele. Hum Mov Sci. 2012;31(6):1670–1687.

[82] Kim YR, Yoo WG. Effects of trajectory exercise using a laser pointer on electromyographic activities of the gluteus maximus and erector spinae during bridging exercises. J Phys Ther Sci. 2016;28(2):632–634.

[83] Clark NC, Röijezon U, Treleaven J. Proprioception in musculoskeletal rehabilitation. Part 2: clinical assessment and intervention. Man Ther. 2015;20(3):378–387.

[84] Borgestig M, Sandqvist J, Ahlsten G, Falkmer T, Hemmingsson H. Gaze-based assistive technology in daily activities in children with severe physical impairments—an intervention study. Dev Neurorehabil. 2016; pp. 1–13. DOI: 10.3109/17518423.2015.1132281

[85] Duchowski AT, Eye Tracking Methodology: Theory and Practise. New York, Springer-Verlag, Inc. 2007, ISBN:1846286085

[86] Ostensjo S, Carlberg EB, Vollestad NK. The use and impact of assistive devices and other environmental modifications on everyday activities and care in young children with cerebral palsy. Disabil Rehabil. 2005;27(14):849–861.

[87] Orlin MN, Palisano RJ, Chiarello LA, Kang LJ, Polansky M, Almasri N, et al. Participation in home, extracurricular, and community activities among children and young people with cerebral palsy. Dev Med Child Neurol. 2010;52(2):160–166.

[88] Sharan D. Functional Outcome of a New Surgical Approach in Severe Cerebral Palsy (GMFCS IV and V), 4th International Cerebral Palsy Conference, Pisa, Italy, October 10–13, 2012.

[89] Rutz E, Tirosh O, Thomason P, Barg A, Graham HK. Stability of the gross motor function classification system after single-event multilevel surgery in children with cerebral palsy. Dev Med Child Neurol. 2012;56:1–5.

[90] Khan MA. Outcome of single-event multilevel surgery in untreated cerebral palsy in a developing country. J Bone Joint Surg Br. 2007;89(8):1088–1091.

[91] Pruitt DW, Tsai T. Common medical comorbidities associated with cerebral palsy. Phys Med Rehabil Clin North Am. 2009;20(3):453–467.

Chapter 8

Assistive and Adaptive Technology in Cerebral Palsy

Alejandro Rafael Garcia Ramirez,
Cleiton Eduardo Saturno, Mauro José Conte,
Jéferson Fernandes da Silva, Mísia Farhat,
Fabiana de Melo Giacomini Garcez Garcez,
Ana Carolina Savall and Elaine Carmelita Piucco

Additional information is available at the end of the chapter

http://dx.doi.org/10.5772/64767

Abstract

Children who suffer from cerebral palsy (CP) face specific challenges, which arise due to motor dysfunction and communication disorders. In some cases, communication is only possible through eye movements and blink, as well as, low amplitude movements of the fingers and toes. Augmentative and alternative communication (AAC) strategies can be used to promote communication in these complex cases. This chapter discusses our experience developing AAC computer's solutions for children with motor and communication disorders. Software and hardware approaches are discussed. This chapter describes solutions developed for desktop computers and mobile devices. These solutions act as complements of therapist's activities, helping disabled people to communicate, and promoting social inclusion.

Keywords: augmentative and alternative communication, cerebral palsy, human-computer interaction

1. Introduction

People with disabilities, such as people who suffer from cerebral palsy (CP), face several challenges in their daily lives. These individuals face specific problems, which arise due to motor dysfunction and communication disorders. These disorders are commonly related to a non-progressive brain damage in early life. CP is also responsible for senses of sight, hearing, speech and language dysfunctions [1].

In addition, cognitive development and communication problems are associated with CP. Like stated in [2], language is affected by brain injury and, therefore, the lack of communication in earlier stages of life can irreversibly impair intellectual ability.

Augmentative and alternative communication (AAC) solutions emerge as solutions to supplement spoken communication or to replace it completely, helping these individuals [3].

AAC solutions can be classified as low-tech or high-tech [2]. The low-tech solutions involve gestures, hand signals and sign language. It also includes the usage of supplementary materials, such as communication boards based on letters, symbols or pictures. It may also be related to picture books, or textured cards using Braille [4].

On the other hand, high-tech solutions involve software and electronic components for standard computers or mobile devices. Dynamic communication displays are examples of high-tech solutions.

However, despite the amount of available technologies, there is not enough guidance available on how to directly collaborate with disabled children and specialists as partners in the design process of assistive technology [5].

This work presents solutions and the methodological aspect of creating, developing and evaluating assistive technologies. These works are based on user centric-design principles [6].

Bibliographic, documentary and experimental research was conducted to achieve our goals. In addition, human-computer solutions designed for severe physical disabilities and lack of speech were studied. The documentary research aimed to analyse the professionals' feedback, verifying the progress using the proposed technologies. On the other hand, the experimental research aimed to use the developed human-computer interfaces, collecting quantitative and qualitative assessments guiding our future works.

2. Assistive technology

Disability is a complex phenomenon, reflected because of the interaction between the individuals and the society in which it lives. It is the result of a deterrent and it can be physical, cognitive, mental, sensory, emotional, developmental, or some combination of these limitations [2]. Disability might be present at birth or arise during life.

Disability is closely related to sensory limitations and emerges when some barriers (physical, communication and information) constrain the participation of individuals in society.

The term "assistive technology" is relatively new and it is used to identify resources, technology and services that contribute to provide or enhance functional abilities of people with disabilities. It includes a wide range of equipment, services and strategies aiming to mitigate the problems faced by individuals with disabilities [2].

In [2], the authors explore the role of assistive technologies in the lives of people with disabilities. They define a HAAT model that means Human Activity Assistive Technology model.

The HAAT model is based on the interaction of four basic components, namely: the activity, the human factor, the assistive technologies and the context in which this interaction occurs (**Figure 1**).

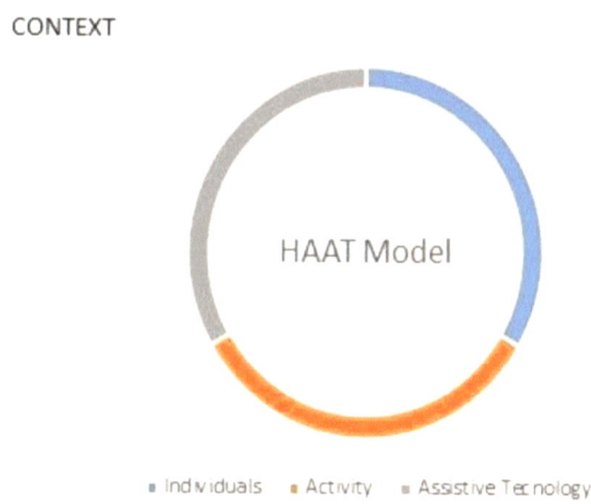

Figure 1. HAAT model. Source: Adapted with permission from [2].

The components of the HAAT model play an important role to understand the methodologies to design assistive technologies. First, a person needs to perform a certain activity, for example, to communicate. In addition, that activity happens in a particular context, for example, in school. For that particular context, and taking into account the activity, may exist an assistive technology that could assist the individual, such as AAC solutions.

The combination between the activity and its context will determine which skills are required to fully realize the activity, so guiding the design of assistive technologies. This model allows understanding the role of assistive technologies, guiding the design process.

3. AAC tool desktop solution

In this section, we describe the solution presented in [7]. The AAC tool solution, as it was named, was based on communication boards and iconographic symbols, commonly found in AAC. It was designed to help the speech therapist intervention. **Figure 3** shows the software interface. The images shown in this figure are merely illustrative.

This interface works as follows. First, a user selects a desired symbol. Next, it is vocalized and, after that, added to the upper left side of the software interface, **Figure 2**. The symbols' library could be customized for each user.

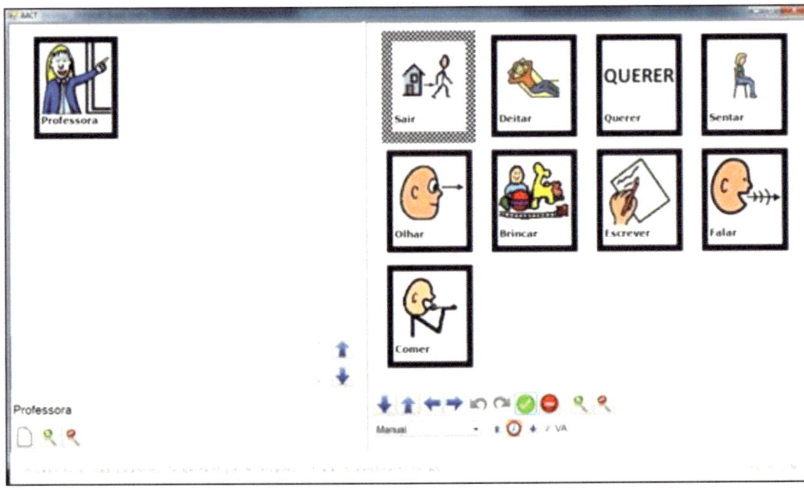

Figure 2. AAC tool desktop interface.

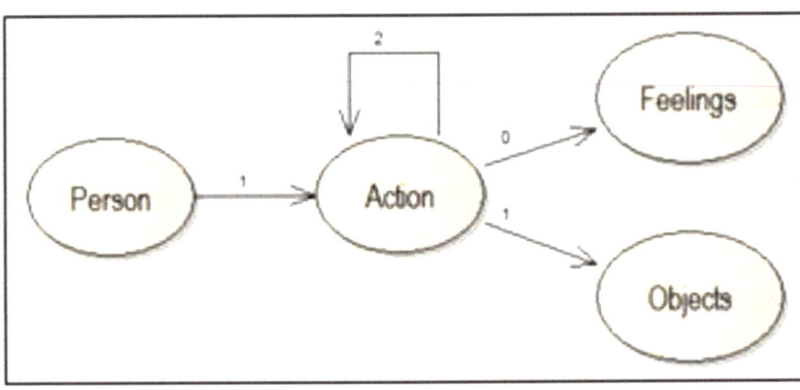

Figure 3. Precedence relationship between symbols and categories.

The software adopts strategies to facilitate the symbols choice. Therefore, symbols commonly used are present first, such as people and greetings. Then, the software suggests other symbols according to the previous ones selected. This feature aims to improve communication speed. Suggestions are based on the previous usage of the tool, and it also depends on the settings performed by the therapist or a caregiver.

It is important to notice that the user could autonomously navigate using the automatic scanning feature, selecting the desired symbols. In addition, the automatic scanning time rate can be settled, according to the users' skills.

The symbols are based on categories, allowing constructing a logical sequence according to the syntax of the user's language (i.e. person, action and feelings). A possible sequence of symbols is based on the syntactic Portuguese language, as illustrated in **Figure 3**.

The software uses the "I + WANT + PLAY" structure, because this grammatical construction is commonly employed by specialists in Brazil. However, some other approaches, for example, based on the verb PLAY + I structure could be used instead.

The tool also features predicting sentences based on graph theory [8]. In addition, it considered important guidelines for human-computer interfaces, adapted from WEB content accessibility guidelines, such as in [7].

This way, pictures have text and oral descriptions. This is very important because CP individuals have difficulties keeping attention on what happens on the computer screen. In addition, the tool lets to resize letters, according to the user's skills, helping to a better understanding of symbols and texts. Border colours and backgrounds are also configurable, according to the user's needs. This is also very important to facilitate symbols recognition.

The buttons located at the bottom right of the software interface emulate mouse and keyboard functions. For this reason, new hardware interfaces could be added without the need to install specific drivers.

Other issues could be conceived, like a vocabulary with numbers and arithmetic operators for a math class or a specific vocabulary for a chemical class containing the elements of the periodic table, for example.

3.1. Evaluation

Students from Special Education Foundation of Santa Catarina—FCEE participated in the study. The volunteers who participated suffer from choreoathetosis, which is a nervous disorder characterized by involuntary and uncontrollable movements. They have preserved the intellectual ability and act as minds trapped into the body [7].

The research sought to analyse the student's performance through a dialogue with and without using the AAC tool. First, the system was presented to the students, enabling them to understand how to use the tool. Then the efficiency and satisfaction using the AAC software were studied.

To evaluate the system, the speech therapist prepared a dialogue, talking about things that are part of the child's routine, such as family, leisure, friends, etc. The speech therapist initiated the dialogue using the low-tech technologies available at FCEE, such as communication boards. In a second stage, the therapist performed the same dialogue but using the software, instead. This procedure was repeated several times, changing the dialogues.

It should be highlighted that the students answered what they want, but it is expected that the answer should be closely related to the one previously given by using the physical board.

Concerning to the hardware resources, students at FCEE commonly use the devices showed in **Figure 4**. Mouse and keyboard devices are commonly used to interact with computers. Besides the usefulness of such suitable devices, they require considerable effort to be actuated and can cause an earlier fatigue.

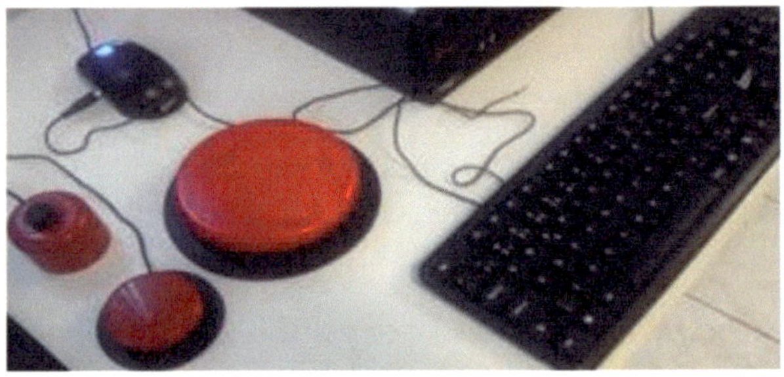

Figure 4. Adapted devices.

Figure 5 shows a stapler device, which was adapted to improve the computer access. The adapted stapler was well suited, because of the shape of the child's hands. It considerably diminishes the spent time to select the symbols on the screen, also reducing the fatigue. This device emulates the click and double clicks functions of the mouse.

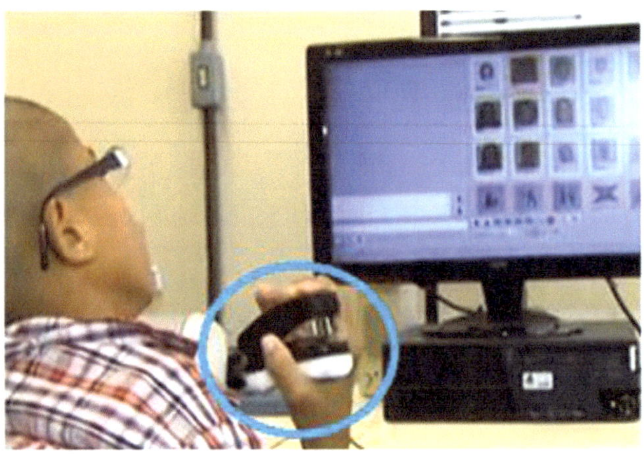

Figure 5. The adapted stapler was a suitable solution.

Symbols selection time rates and errors committed were computed. Typically, students attempt an average rate of 15 symbols selections per minute, when using low-tech communication boards. When using the system, those rates were worse, even though, on several occasions, the students achieved similar result. In addition, sometimes no coherent phrases were constructed, but it was observed that error rates gradually decrease with the usage of the interface [7].

In addition, an evaluation was carried out to demonstrate the symbol prediction feature, which is based on previous symbols selections. The goal was to build a phrase and to repeat it several times. Then the spent time to construct each phrase was verified. The tests used an automatic scanning rate of 1 s. **Figure 6** shows that it is possible to decrease the time required to construct new phrases.

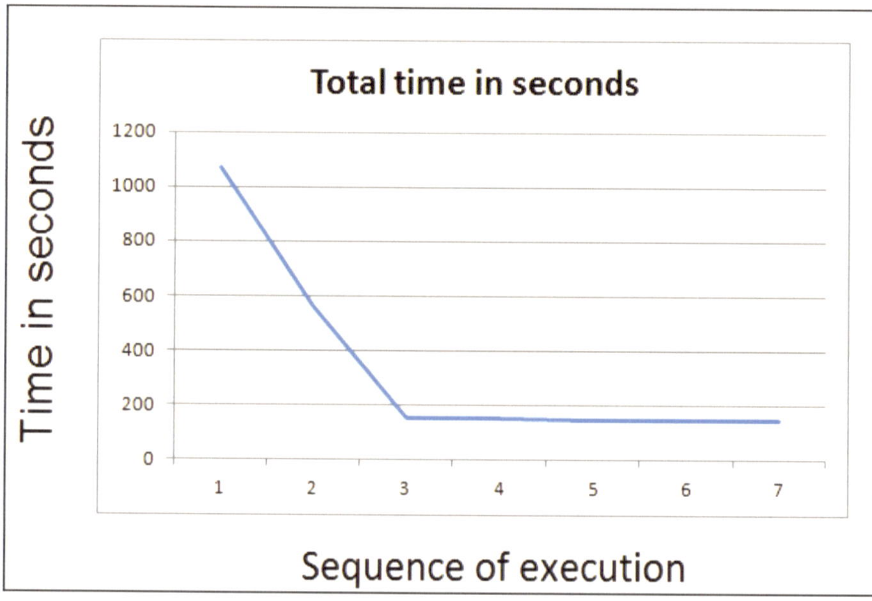

Figure 6. Performance of the symbol prediction feature.

In addition, speech therapists at FCEE performed qualitative assessments. Interviews evaluate issues related to student's behaviour and performance. Aspects such as simplicity, software interaction, configurability, images quality, screen navigation resources and students' evolution were evaluated as good, following the recommendations in [9].

The specialists conclude that it is easy to understand the operation and principles of the tool. In addition, according to [7], "they registered that a more efficient interaction with the software will be directly related to the complexity of the student needs and, according to their opinion, this represents the greatest challenge".

This software is opened to developers and can be accessed at https://sourceforge.net/projects/aact/?source=navbar [Accessed: March 26, 2016].

4. AAC mobile solution

After developing the AAC solution for desktops, we think about enhancing the same idea to tablets, applying the solution at Association of Parents and Friends of Exceptional Children (APAE). This section discusses our experience developing the AAC solution for mobile devices.

The problem faced at APAE is that the students with CP also suffer from severe intellectual disability. Therefore, the software AAC tool, developed for desktops, was useless in that context.

For this reason, we redirect our proposal, guided by the HAAT model. Then, a new tool for mobile devices interaction focusing users having intellectual disabilities was designed. The solution concerned about the presentation and organization of content based on accessibility standards [9].

It is worth noting that the development considered accessibility recommendations, according to the W3C Group, July 9, 2009, in particular, the Mobile Web Best Practices (MWBP) [10].

4.1. Interface

The new software guides the work of professionals at APAE. It was designed as an educational strategy, contributing, booth, as a tool to study the intellectual disability and as an AAC strategy.

The app is not by itself decisive to diagnostic a sort of intellectual disability, but it helps in the professional's decision. It should be used along with other international validated tools and theoretical references founded at Diagnostic and Statistical Manual of Mental Disorders (DSM) [11] and American Association of Intellectual Disability (AAIDI), for example.

Figure 7 shows the initial screen. In order to login, the professional informs its identification and a password. Selecting the "keep connected" option, the specialist may choose to store the password, so that it will no longer be necessary to re-enter it in future accesses.

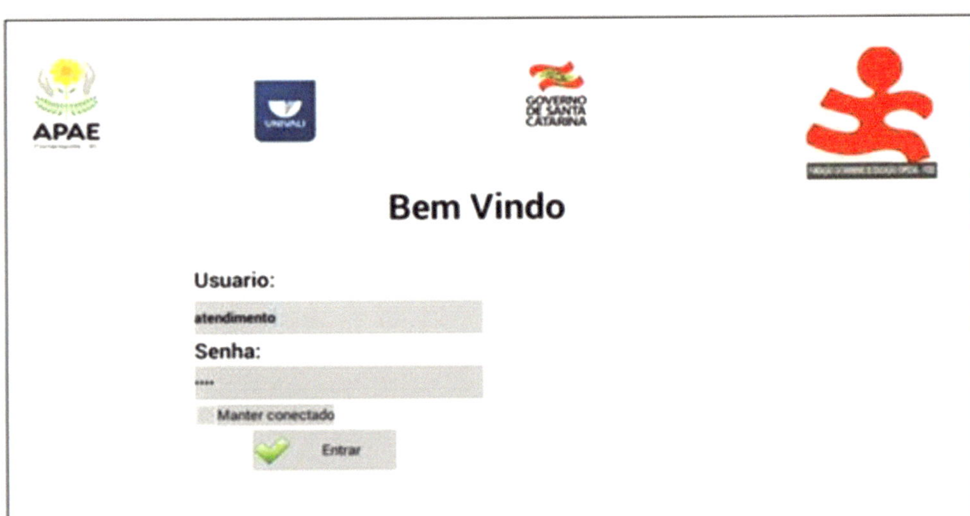

Figure 7. Welcome screen.

When accessing the system, the specialist can create and configure the student profile (**Figure 8**). It is important to notice that the database involves personal data, so it must be treated with all the necessary integrity and security.

http://dx.doi.org/10.5772/64767

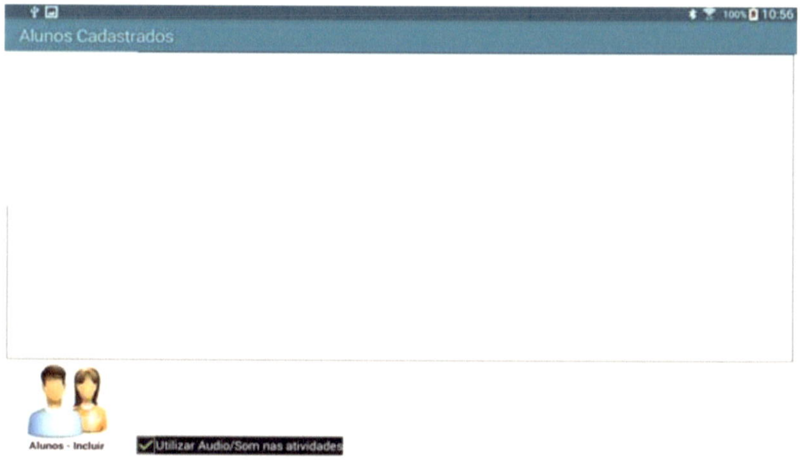

Figure 8. Students profile.

The main activity conceived for this app is to study the student's cognitive ability. This is done by selecting and grouping symbols from different categories such as clothing, food, animals, transportation, etc., grouping them according to their relationship within each category.

Before this app, the students had to select, by hand, symbols and context cards randomly spread in a round table. This made the task of selecting them difficult for CP users.

Figure 9 shows the default categories and symbols configured for this app. The professionals at APAE could add new categories and symbols. In this screen, the student's name can be heard through the speakers.

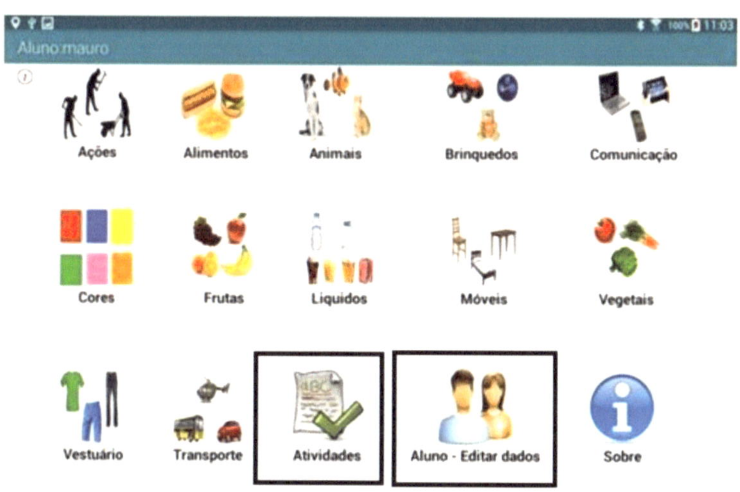

Figure 9. Categories and symbols.

Actions, foods, animals, toys, communication devices, colours, fruits, liquid foods, furniture, vegetables, clothing and means of transportation are the chosen categories (**Figure 9**). In **Figure 8**, a link to the student profile and activities was highlighted in black squares.

The About option, located at the bottom in **Figure 9**, gives information about the student, the APAE professionals and the institutions who collaborate with this research. It is important to remark that all the symbols, feedbacks, texts and sounds can be configured by the professionals.

Figure 10 shows the main activity conceived for this app, named Drag and Drop. The main purpose of this activity is to test the cognitive ability of the student by selecting symbols from different categories such as clothing, food, animals, etc., grouping them according to their relationship within each category.

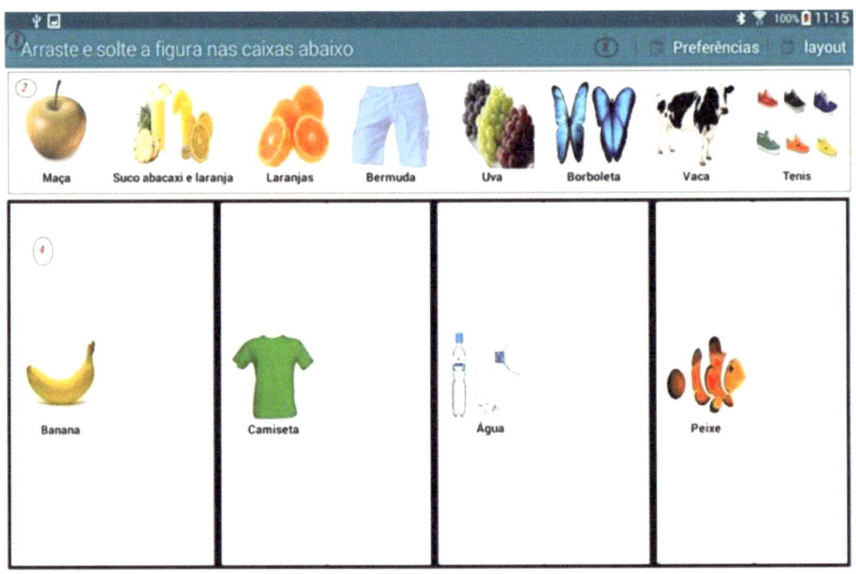

Figure 10. Symbols and the related categories in the Drag and Drop activity.

When performing this activity, the student should drag the symbols from different categories, pictured at the top of the screen, dropping them inside the boxes that appear in the lower part of the screen. To this end, the app uses the touch feature, commonly available in mobile devices.

The professionals can configure both the symbols shown at the top of the screen and the symbols that appear at the bottom of the screen. At the end of this activity, the symbols are properly grouped into their respective categories, or not. This test contributes to evaluate intellectual disability.

Figure 11 shows the symbols used in the Foods category. An auditory feedback can be associated to each symbol.

http://dx.doi.org/10.5772/64767

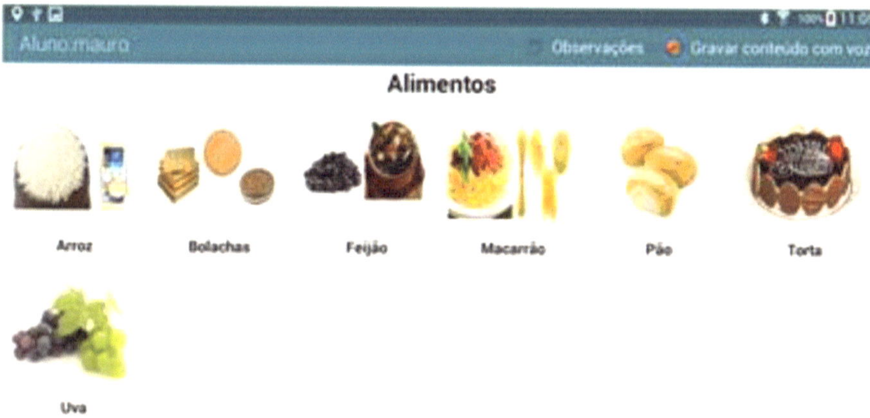

Figure 11. Symbols related to the Foods category.

Figure 12 shows an activity specially conceived for CP users. This activity was named Hit the Target and aims to analyse the motor skills of the student.

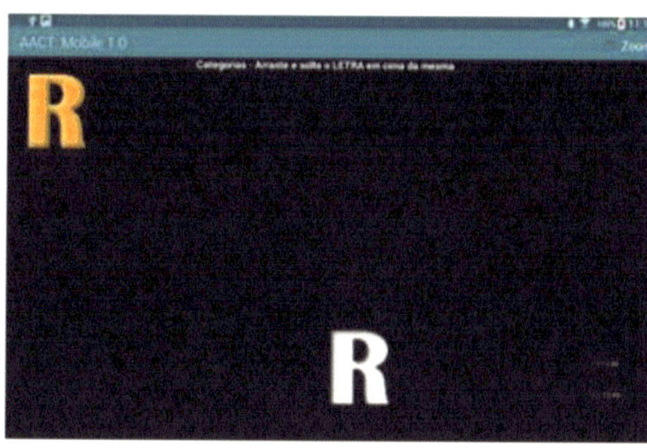

Figure 12. Hit the Target activity.

The goal of this activity is to measure the time the user spent to select the letter at the upper left of the screen, hitting the same letter at the lower centre of the screen.

To this end it was used the Touch Listener feature in the Android operating system [12]. The Touch Listener feature allows the programmer to create new functions for each move classification, which are then processed whenever a movement event occurs. Among them are the touch itself, identified by the action ACTION_DOWN code and dragging, identified by ACTION_MOVE code.

These data may subsequently be considered in the Drag and Drop activity in order to allow users with motor disorders use the application with autonomy.

Figure 13 shows other kind of activities that can be done using the app. In this case, a speech therapist can work with isolated symbols to develop speech and auditory cognitive abilities, such as in speech therapy sessions, for example. It should be remarked that new symbols and sounds could be included or configured to attend users in different situations.

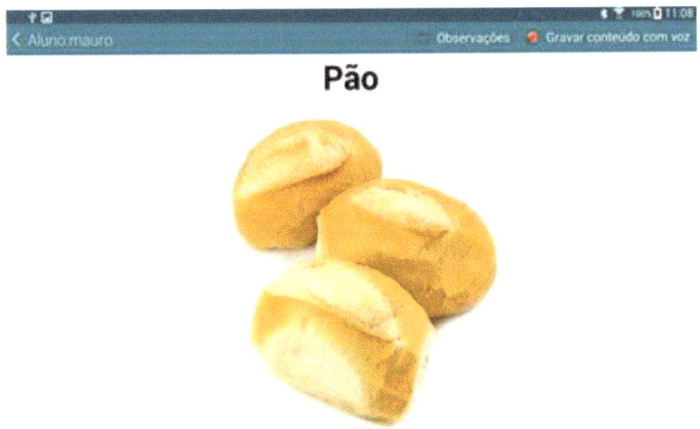

Figure 13. Working with the Foods category.

4.2. Evaluation

Nowadays, the app is being evaluated at APAE, using the system usability scale (SUS) questionnaire [13]. The APAE specialists are registering their perception about the student's performance using the tool. The SUS will highlight the positives and negatives aspects of the system.

According to [13], (at least) ten statements, being evaluated on a scale from 1 to 5, should compose the survey by establishing a balance between positive and negative assertions. "The Software operation is simple" and "The Software often induce errors" are examples of these assertions.

Other assertions are related to the complexity and, confidence using the system, and other usability issues. This questionnaire is under evaluation at APAE.

The app will indicate the degree of physical and cognitive involvement of each child, computing separately the questionnaires and grouping them according to similar cognitive and motor skills.

Preliminary evaluation shows the following contributions: easy handling application, good images contrast, easy calibration and automatic adjust of the touch screen time; useful for AAC; several language stimulation possibilities, including voice recording; and rich in visual stimuli.

Still, we have to improve images resolution, enhance the resources for speech therapy activities and insert new basic functions of the language.

The AAC mobile software is also opened to developers and can be accessed at https://sourceforge.net/projects/aact-mobile/?source=navbar [Accessed: March 26, 2016].

5. New study

A new study is being performed using a brain-computer interface (BCI) [14]. The development is based on the Emotiv Epoc [15]. In particular, we are using EEG signals [16]. This new user-computer interaction is being integrated with the two software solutions previously described, emulating mouse and keyboard commands.

At this moment, a software pilot solution was designed to test the computer interaction with CP individuals (**Figure 14**). Our goal is to find metrics, such as success, errors, time rates, number of phrases construction, satisfaction and others parameters that will be identified when performing the next stages of this research.

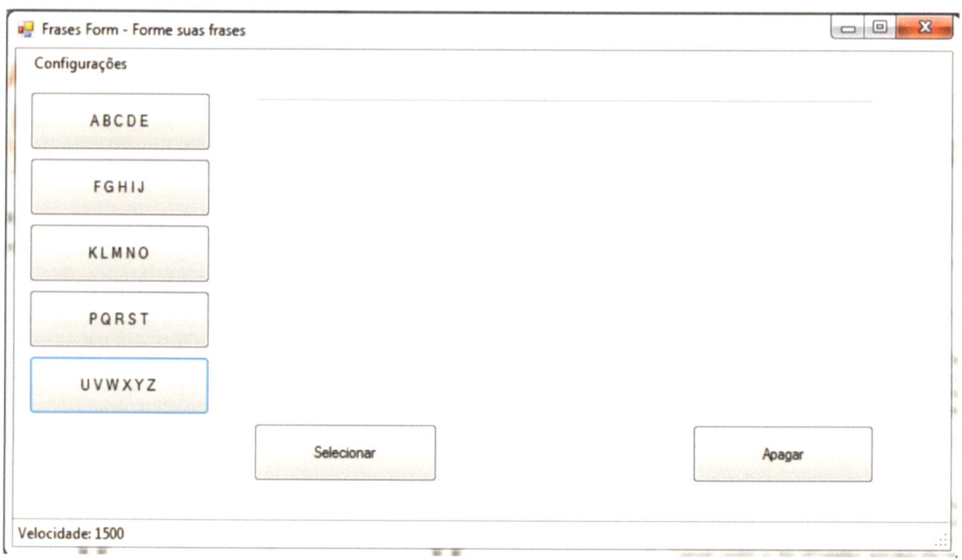

Figure 14. PhraseForm software interface.

The PhraseForm software validates the basic headset functions of the Emotiv Epoc SDK (Software Development Kit). The SDK links users and the Emotiv Epoc, processing the electrical signals coming from the headset. The PhraseForm software emulates mouse and keyboard commands, as delete or line break, for example, also selecting characters on the screen in order to form sentences.

The software looks for the best actions to be captured using the EEG signals. Based on this interface, the BCI technique is being validated by CP individuals.

Figure 14 shows the FraseForm user-application interface. Actions such as blink, show teeth, eyebrow, frowning, laugh, neutral, smile, etc., could be configured to interact with the software, selecting or deleting characters. Speech therapist is guiding the process of select the best actions choice for each student.

Nowadays this study is performed at FCEE. Preliminary results promise the access to computer resources with autonomy by CP individuals. **Figure 15** shows a CP volunteer using the system.

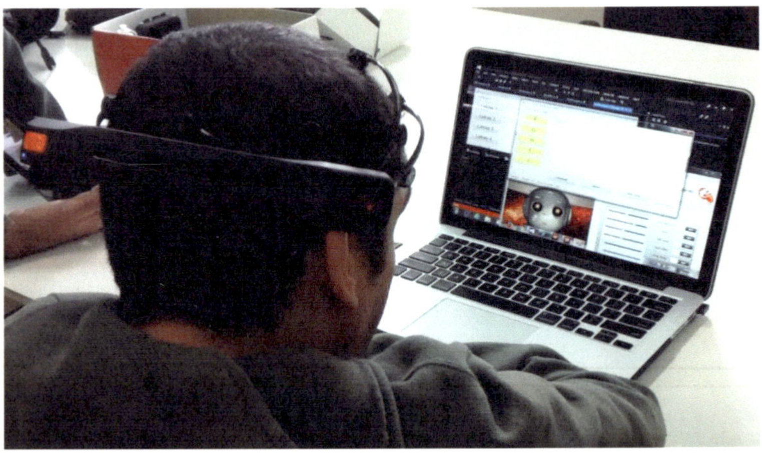

Figure 15. CP volunteer testing the BCI.

6. Conclusions

This work discusses our experience developing AAC solutions for students with motor and communication disorders, which is commonly found in cases of cerebral palsy. The students attend the Special Education Foundation of Santa Catarina—FCEE and Association of Parents and Friends of Exceptional Children (APAE) in Brazil.

Our first experience was developed at FCEE. The AAC tool solution features characteristics that are considered relevant to the design of AAC systems. It considered several recommended guidelines to develop human-computer interfaces, adapted from WEB content accessibility.

Using the software, symbols can be selected from a pre-configured vocabulary, inserting them in a designated area. Phrases constructions are based on symbols and their respective categories. This allows mounting a logical sequence according to the syntax of the user's language. We adopt a sequence based on syntactic Portuguese language. Iconographic symbols convey needs, wishes, desires and ideas.

http://dx.doi.org/10.5772/64767

The study validates symbol suggestion features, demonstrating the efficiency of this approach for assisting sentences construction. There are also presented qualitative assessments from speech therapists.

The second study was developed at APAE, together with the professionals and students who attend this institution. Educators, speech therapists, psychologists and occupational therapists took part in this new study.

The app features an alternative and augmentative communication tool for children having CP, but not restricted to this public. The solution was designed to assist professionals who act in special education assessing the intellectual disability. The app is based on the MWBP accessibility recommendations.

The AAC mobile supports the assessment of students with suspected disabilities. It encompasses various activities/strategies within just one application. It also explores basic functions of language and its categories such as colours, animals and everyday objects, for example, contributing to the speech therapy.

The evaluation process using the system usability scale (SUS) is still under construction, but preliminary results showed its usefulness to study the intellectual disability, which is also useful as an alternative and augmentative communication tool.

This app cannot be considered, by itself, as the only key to diagnose intellectual disability, because there are internationally validated tools to this end. Instead, it configures a new way to interact with children with CP using the technological advances. Nowadays, we are studying new ways of interaction with computers and mobile devices using eye tracking and electroencephalography.

This research deals with a set of accessibility guidelines that benefit researchers and practitioners, giving more evidence about the design of AAC computer-based solutions for people with limited speech or language skills, who are the centre of these solutions. In this work, the HAAT model guides the design of such assistive resources.

Preliminary results in this field promise alternative ways to access computer resources, promoting autonomy, giving more evidence about the design of AAC computer and hardware-based solutions devoted to people having reduced language skills and motor disorders. It is important to remark that the AAC tools we presented are intended to be used in the school, according to the ethics protocol of this research.

Acknowledgements

The National Council of Scientific and Technological Development (CNPq) support this research under the 458672 process. In addition, the Foundation for Supporting Research and Innovation in Santa Catarina (FAPESC) supported this research under grant 2015TR300. It is also been covered by the Ethics Committee on Human Research.

Author details

Alejandro Rafael Garcia Ramirez[1*], Cleiton Eduardo Saturno[1], Mauro José Conte[1], Jéferson Fernandes da Silva[1], Mísia Farhat[2], Fabiana de Melo Giacomini Garcez Garcez[3], Ana Carolina Savall[2] and Elaine Carmelita Piucco[2]

*Address all correspondence to: garcia.ramirez@gmail.com

1 Applied Computing Department, University of Vale de Itajaí, Itajaí, Brazil

2 Assistive Technology Department, Foundation for Special Education in Santa Catarina – FCEE, São José, Brazil

3 Augmentative and Alternative Communication Department, Association of Parents and Friends of Exceptional Children, Florianópolis, Brazil

References

[1] S. Levitt. O tratamento da paralisia cerebral e do retardo motor (The treatment of cerebral palsy and motor disorders). 1st ed. São Paulo: Manole; 2011.

[2] A. M. Cook, J. M. Polgar. Cook & Hussey's, Assistive Technologies: Principles and Practice. 3er ed. USA: Mosby Elsevier; 2013. 496 p.

[3] O. C. Ann, L. B. Theng. Biometrics based assistive communication tool for children with special needs. In: 7th International Conference on Information Technology; 12–13 July; Kuching, Sarawak. 2011. p. 1-6. DOI: 10.1109/CITA.2011.5999527

[4] J. Sigafoos, R. W. Schlosser. Dean Sutherland. Augmentative and Alternative Communication [Internet]. 2010. Available from: http://cirrie.buffalo.edu/encyclopedia/en/article/50/ [Accessed: March 26, 2016]

[5] A. J. Hornof. Designing with children with severe motor impairments. In: ACM CHI Conference on Human Factors in Computing Systems; April 9th; Boston, USA. ACM Press; 2009. p. 2177-62180.

[6] T. Lowdermilk. User-Centered Design: A Developer's Guide to Building User-Friendly Applications. 1st ed. USA: O'Reilly Media; 2013. 154 p.

[7] C. E. Saturno, M. Farhat, M. J. Conte, E. C. Piucco, A. R. G. Ramirez. An augmentative and alternative communication tool for children and adolescents with cerebral palsy. Behaviour & Information Technology 2015;34(6):632-645. DOI: 10.1080/0144929X.2015.1019567

[8] K. Ruohonen. Graph Theory. [online]. 2013. Available from: http://math.tut.fi/~ruohonen/GT_English.pdf [Accessed: May 01, 2014].

[9] W. Albert, T. Tullis. Measuring the User Experience. 2nd ed. USA: Elsevier Inc; 2013. 300 p. DOI: 10.1016/B978-0-12-415781-1.00013-3

[10] J. Rabin, C. Mccathienevile. Mobile Web Best Practices 1.0.W3C [Internet]. 2008. Available from: http:// Www.W3.Org/Tr/Mobile-Bp/ [Accessed: March 26, 2016]

[11] American Psychiatric Association. Diagnostic and Statistical Manual of Mental Disorders [Internet]. 2014. Available from: http://c026204.cdn.sapo.io/1/c026204/cld-file/1426522730/6d77c9965e17b15/b37dfc58aad8cd477904b9bb2ba8a75b/obaudoedu-cador/2015/DSM%20V.pdf [Accessed: March 26, 2016]

[12] J. R. Lewis. IBM computer usability satisfaction questionnaires: psychometric evaluation and instructions for use. International Journal of Human-Computer Interaction 1995;7(1):57-58. DOI: 10.1080/10447319509526110

[13] N. Smyth. Android Studio Development Essentials. 2015. eBookFrency.

[14] B. Grainmann, B. Allison, G. Pfurtscheller (eds.), Brain–computer Interfaces: a gentle introduction. *Brain–computer Interfaces*. The Frontiers Collection, DOI 10.1007/978-3-642-02091-9_1, Springer-Verlag Berlin Heidelberg; 2010.

[15] Emotiv Epoc. http://emotiv.com/epoc/. [March 26, 2016{/Date Accessed].

[16] M. Poulos. On the use of EEG features towards person identification via neural networks. Medical Informatics and the Internet in Medicine 1999;26(1):35-48.